MW00811315

"If you give your body what it requires to slow the aging process, it provides the wisdom and science discussed in this excellent book."

—MARK C. HOUSTON, MD, MS, MSC
AUTHOR OF *THE TRUTH ABOUT HEART DISEASE AND CONTROLLING HIGH BLOOD PRESSURE*

RESTORE

RESTORE

OPTIMAL HEALTH THROUGH
BIOIDENTICAL HORMONES

GREG BRANNON
MD, FACOG, ABAARM

Advantage | Books

Published by Advantage Books, Charleston, South Carolina.
An imprint of Advantage Media.

ADVANTAGE is a registered trademark, and the Advantage colophon is a trademark of Advantage Media Group, Inc.

Printed in the United States of America.

10 9 8 7 6 5 4 3 2 1

ISBN: 978-1-64225-750-2 (Hardcover)
ISBN: 978-1-64225-749-6 (eBook)

Library of Congress Control Number: 2023921722

Cover and layout design by Lance Buckley

Scripture quotations taken from the (NASB®) New American Standard Bible®, Copyright © 1960, 1971, 1977, 1995, 2020 by The Lockman Foundation. Used by permission. All rights reserved. lockman.org

This publication is designed to provide accurate and authoritative information in regard to the subject matter covered. It is sold with the understanding that the publisher is not engaged in rendering legal, accounting, or other professional services. If legal advice or other expert assistance is required, the services of a competent professional person should be sought.

Advantage Books is an imprint of Advantage Media Group. Advantage Media helps busy entrepreneurs, CEOs, and leaders write and publish a book to grow their business and become the authority in their field. Advantage authors comprise an exclusive community of industry professionals, idea-makers, and thought leaders. For more information go to **advantagemedia.com**.

Disclaimer

This book is based on research and contains the opinions and ideas of the author. It contains advice and information relating to healthcare. It should be used as a supplement rather than to replace the advice of your doctor or other licensed healthcare professional.

It is intended to provide helpful and informative materials on the medical subjects in the publication. It is sold with the understanding that the author and publisher are not engaged in rendering health, medical, or other professional advice to the individual reader. The reader should not use the information within as a substitute for the advice of their doctor or other licensed healthcare providers.

To the best of the author's knowledge, the information provided is accurate at the time of publication.

The author and publisher disclaim any liability whatsoever concerning any loss, injury, or damage arising directly or indirectly from the use of this book

Dedication

"A journey of a thousand miles begins with a single step" is a saying by an ancient Chinese philosopher. The original text is "A journey of a thousand *li* starts beneath one's feet.'" Here, *li* means distance. This quote was first used in the Chinese classic text the *Tao Te Ching*, attributed to Lao Tzu, a renowned Chinese philosopher. It was probably written between the fourth and sixth centuries.[1]

This journey has been remarkable. But more than remarkable has been my best friend, the mother of our seven beautiful children, my love, my bride—Jody. We would not be at this magic inflection point without her devotion and commitment. She has been side by side with me for every step of the journey, and her deep belief in our work has driven us forward every day.

I dedicate this book to Jody Brannon.

> *And the Lord God fashioned into a woman the rib*
> *which He had taken from the man,*
> *and brought her to the man.*
> *Then the man said,*
> *"At last this is bone of my bones,*
> *and flesh of my flesh;*
> *She shall be called 'woman,'*
> *because she was taken out of man."*
> *For this reason,*
> *a man shall leave his father and his mother,*
> *and be joined to his wife;*
> *and they shall become one flesh.*
> *And the man and his wife were both naked,*
> *but they were not ashamed.*

GENESIS 2:22-25

Foreword

Imagine getting a troubling health diagnosis. You're suddenly facing a life that looks nothing like you'd planned it. Your treatments will disrupt your routines. You won't feel as energetic as you used to. You might not even be able to continue doing the work you've done for years.

Some people in this situation will tackle the new challenge with urgency. They'll do the treatments, make the changes, and adapt to their new realities. Other people will deny the diagnosis and won't be willing to fight the disease because they don't want to disrupt the life they've become comfortable with.

They continue as-is, thinking they're maintaining a status quo that they find acceptable.

But what they don't see is that the disease is already changing that status quo for them. Rather than create the opportunity to shape their new reality themselves, they are surrendering influence over their future by not accepting what's really happening.

This is where the entire healthcare industry is today, and this is the wake-up call that Dr. Greg Brannon has enlightened us all to see with the opportunity to seize in this book, *Restore*.

*It's becoming less about the business defining the individual,
and much more about the individual defining the business.*

I made this declaration in my 2017 book, *The Innovation Mentality*. What did this statement mean? That corporate America, higher education, and healthcare institutions were in the process of losing their ability to control what should matter to the individual. Having interviewed hundreds of these institutions' leaders in my Forbes.com column, most leaders couldn't see the significance of this shift (from institution to individual). And for those that could see it, they kept quiet knowing this would reveal their own obsolescence. My message to these institutions' leaders: we must shift from ruling by standardization to leading with personalization.

To further elevate the sense of urgency for those institutions and their physicians, deans, and presidents I published my 2019 book, *Leadership in the Age of Personalization: Why Standardization Fails in the Age of Me*. This manifesto was my attempt to create a clarion call to disrupt the status quo that only knew how to approach innovation, growth, and opportunities based on old, outdated standards that didn't account enough for what mattered to the individual. It was an effort to help these physicians, deans, and presidents see and understand "the troubling health diagnosis" and how to interrupt and pivot their thinking to accept the changing world around them that would redefine leadership and profitability. It was still difficult for these institutions' leaders to see this new reality while their organizations were enjoying (short-term) success and profitability, by doing things the way they'd always done them. But the era of personalization started to catch wind when the pandemic shook the world in 2020 and the limitations of standardization were finally revealed.

I've learned many things the hard way about institutional leaders, but the following statement stands out from the rest: knowing what's right, isn't enough to start doing what's right, and knowing something's wrong isn't enough to stop doing it. Physicians, deans, and presidents don't want to be accountable to accept new realities, so they create their own. They become skeptical and ignore it until one of their competitors does it first or when a global pandemic forces it upon them (i.e., telehealth, virtual education, remote working, etc.). And throughout the process of being hopeful that institutions will eventually do what's right, millions of people are suppressed, and they sacrifice their own dignity out of the fear of doing what's right.

Dr. Greg Brannon is inviting us all to reclaim our dignity. He is helping us understand that if we are going to live our best lives, we must embrace our freedom and liberty. Dr. Brannon is teaching a lesson about having the courage to do what's right for our body, mind, and soul so that we can encourage others to do the same.

In the midst of the pandemic, Wall Street Analysis' RBC Capital Markets issued a report in November 2021 (RBC Imagine™ Preparing for Hyperdrive) declaring an "individual revolution"—saying that the balance of power is shifting away from traditional institutions into the hands of individuals. The report states, "This will create a new world order in every aspect of the global economy and will likely be the single biggest disruptive force to existing centers of power."[2]

This new era of personalization was finally seen and understood not only because of this report but also the aftermath of the pandemic including but not limited to nursing shortages in hospitals due to poor working conditions, the Great Resignation in corporate America, and the significant declines in university enrollment. These actions would not only awaken institutional leaders and the investor community but would also give me the leverage needed to take my manifesto to the next level in my 2022 book, Unleashing Individuality which featured revealing research about the lack of resilience and reinvention readiness to embrace today's age of personalization. The book would also outline how to capitalize on this new era of personalization that is redefining the ways we work, lead, live, conduct business, and achieve financial success and significance.

For example, in healthcare, it's about seeing and treating patients as individuals. This is achieved when people know they matter and have the option to choose what is in their best interest. At a larger scale, it is the act of adapting the way an organization or industry functions to make it more likely that both internal and external constituencies at all levels build the skills, have the tools, and provide options to serve, see, and treat people as individuals.

Dr. Brannon teaches us through his pioneering and groundbreaking work in bioidentical hormone replacement therapies (BHRT), about the many barriers to personalization that exist within the healthcare system because it's designed to do what is in the best interest of the organization, not the individual. For example, healthcare leaders tend to view patients and employees as either health experts or not (with a medical, nursing, pharmacy degree or not), rather than as a person with experience and insights that might be relevant, whether or not they have a degree—even in situations where a degree is not necessary. Patients are often seen in terms of their disease category (i.e., cancer patient) rather than as the individuals they are, which can significantly affect their experiences while receiving care.

Breaking decades of attitudes and behaviors that are deeply ingrained in the healthcare system can be overwhelming. Dehumanizing behaviors arose for a reason: they were a way for a large system to create order and efficiency at the expense of what matters to individuals and their healthcare goals. For example, one of the major hurdles we face in healthcare is the current payer (insurance) reimbursement model. Rather than prioritizing health and wellness, which is what most individuals truly desire, our system focuses on compensating for sick care and medical procedures. It's disheartening that organizations are rewarded for replacing hips rather than helping individuals achieve weight loss or overall well-being. What complicates the issue is the lack of effective systems to understand what truly matters to patients. As a result, we often find ourselves delivering care based on the healthcare systems' notions of quality and value instead of aligning with the patients' priorities during a specific moment in their lives.

Dr. Brannon challenges us all to reflect and evaluate what matters to us as individuals and the freedom we possess to control our health and well-being to make the most of this one precious life we have. Restore is not only a book about the life-changing advancements of BHRT and aging gracefully but also about taking control of your life for the betterment of a healthier whole.

As a patient of Dr. Brannon's, I can personally attest to the remarkable journey he is taking us on.

Glenn Llopis
CEO at Glenn Llopis Group (GLLG)
Founder of the Leadership in the Age of Personalization Movement
www.ageofpersonalization.com

Contents

PREFACE:
We're Not The First 1

INTRODUCTION:
"The Game Is Afoot!" 7

CHAPTER 1:
Chasing the Dream for Centuries 17

CHAPTER 2:
Pinch Yourself—You May Now Restore Your Body Chemistry 29

CHAPTER 3:
Understanding Your Hormones—The Energy Sources for Your Body 63

CHAPTER 4:
Medical Liberty Is a Verb—How Well-Intended Ideas Become Stupid Rules 79

The Miracle of Our Hormones 121

CHAPTER 5:
Women's Lifetime of Choices for Optimal Health—
It's Much More Than Estrogen 147

CHAPTER 6:

**Men's Lifetime of Choices for Optimal Health—
It's Much More Than Testosterone** 189

CHAPTER 7:

**Optimal Wellness—Your Wellness Journey
After Your First Hormone Replacement** 227

CHAPTER 8:

**The Magnificent Role of Nutrition in Quality of Life—
Fasting, Peptides, and Making Good Choices** 283

The Costs and Minor Side Effects of BHRT 313

CHAPTER 9:

There's Never Been a Time Like This in Human Health 323

Other Books and Research to Inspire You 331

Acknowledgments 339

PREFACE

We're Not the First

From the dawn of time, humans could be sure of two things. Most men and women would experience the exuberance and invulnerability of being young. In the Middle Ages, young men trained for a pugilistic life and watched their fathers ride off to noble battles. *Strong. Purposeful. Modeling a set of moral virtues.* These young men were eager to become knights. Young women gained incredible strength, preparing to become a parent, inspire the family, and guard the home front.

The second revelation was a slow realization that the body relentlessly declines with aging.

As Kate Wong, a senior editor of *Scientific American*, once wrote: "For most of human evolution, our ancestors mostly lived fast and died young."[3]

"The trend of having a low life expectancy at birth and a significantly higher life expectancy during adulthood continued into the Middle Ages. As the *BBC* reported, the life expectancy at birth for males born between 1276 and 1300 was just over 31 years. But for those who reached age 20, it jumped to 45 years. And if they reached 30, living into their fifties became likely," noted a scholarly article on the MassMutual website "Age Up."

Nothing could be done about it except perhaps, if maybe—just maybe—the legends were true. Could it be that there really is a Holy Grail, a vessel that may carry the elixir of eternal health or long life? Some believed that the grail is the philosopher's stone, a stone that can give longevity. Or perhaps it also played into the fountain-of-youth narrative that later involved historical conquests. Other myths have attributed the Holy Grail to satisfying the needs of whoever drank from it by providing a deeply spiritual or mystical experience.

They served their king. They served their church. And along the way to fulfilling their destiny, they rode out to seek the Holy Grail or the Fountain of Youth. Their quests have continually been passed down through legends and storytelling, even to our lifetimes. They sought the miracle to restore their wellness and believed an answer was out there.

So this generation is one of many to seek a remedy for the inevitable aging decline. It's something our ancestors deeply longed for—a restoration. People have hoped for this for centuries on every continent. Many chased the dream. What were they thinking? What starts a pilgrimage? Some sought everlasting life. Most were looking for healing, a renewal of youthfulness, or an absence of suffering and decline. Evildoers sought these things to obtain unspeakable power.

During his twilight years, American author Mark Twain noted that "life would be infinitely happier if we could only be born at the age of eighty and gradually approach eighteen."[4]

Twain's quip was only one of many complaints about aging recorded for as long as humans have dreaded the downside of a long life. The ancient Greek poet Homer called old age "loathsome," and William Shakespeare termed it a "hideous winter."[5]

No longer do we have to surrender to the harmful effects of aging without a fight. This is a big moment. Do I sound excited? You bet.

The Holy Grail that we refer to in *Restore* is not the precious cup of Christ. People still eagerly seek that around the world. Our grail represents the crusading advancement of science, which has now arrived at the point where we can experience new wellness even into advanced aging.

Today, our crusading knights are the physicians and researchers who have kept sight of the quest. They have devised a remedy to enable us all to age gracefully and miraculously.

Decades from now, hormone restoration will be commonplace. It will not seem miraculous, and people will scratch their heads about why it took us so long to figure this out.

The centuries-long quest has paused here, in this time and place. Answers have been found. Medical science takes time, and that time has proven that this can be done safely and with few side effects. Our energies and body systems can be renewed now. It's not a dream. It's here.

The goal of reversing the inevitable decline in our health has become a reality. It's called bioidentical hormone replacement therapy (BHRT). I have provided this medical treatment for over twenty thousand patients with no complications for over a decade. I use the breakthrough technology of natural, holistic, subcutaneous pellets that dissolve over time, restoring our hormones to optimal levels.

We can restore the wellness of our bodies, taking advantage of our wisdom to age gracefully. Culturally, this means that our useful, productive lives will be extended, and we can avoid the atrophy of frail old age. This enormously impacts our nation's healthcare system and how we view prevention.

Restore contains the science and methodology for you to do so. This new field of restorative medicine has evolved rapidly in the last ten years. Millions of people have experienced this renewal.

The breakthrough came when our scientists created a natural, bioidentical, holistic way to do this. *Integrative Medicine, A Clinician's Journal* describes restorative medicine as focusing on the importance of a balanced endocrine system by recognizing how chemical messengers influence each other. Stabilizing the endocrine system, rather than treating a single hormone, helps optimize health and promote longevity. Restorative medicine aims to reduce or eliminate the need for ongoing medical treatment, when possible, by truly restoring health at its core.[6]

We have brooded about becoming old, frail, helpless, weak, and dependent for our entire lives. It's hard to let that go. *Nothing we can do about it. It's normal.* It's not normal anymore. We no longer must surrender to the harmful effects of aging without a fight. We no longer must surrender our wisdom as our brain cells struggle with the agony of dementia. This is a big moment. How about having all your mental faculties in place, and a healthy body, for your entire life span?

If you could go back in time, what would you say to your twenty-five-year-old self? Through the power of BHRT, you can now say, "Relax. I will not allow my hormones to become depleted as I age. I will keep my fully functional brain throughout my life without dementia and strong bones and muscles. I will enjoy my life with the benefit of having no diabetes, no hypertension, healthy body chemistry, and all the energy I need to enjoy every minute of this precious life I have been given."

We are emerging from the pandemic years of mass death, illness, uncertainty, and social disarray; many of us may feel skeptical when something this good—and this powerful—comes along. The cloud has lifted, and somehow the gatekeepers of our malaise lost their nerve and allowed this to pass.

But we understand the words "scientific discovery" that held such positive meaning during the 2020 pandemic.

Our ancestors prepared the ground for this future, and their quests have led to the present clinical advances. It has not been a single knight who made these victories. Thousands of knights in a medical army all over the world accumulated their wisdom and their evidence. Our quest has resulted in this significant holistic breakthrough in restoring our wellness as we age.

And it has been a quest. Decades ago, millions of women were prescribed hormone therapy through hormones created from the urine of pregnant horses to combat menopause.

And while this was going on, progressive scientists and physicians began their own quest. They gathered and started studying the power of hormone replacement, comparing notes. They embarked upon a quest to seek something better, something gentler on the body, something more natural. Then, like Sherlock Holmes revealing new clues, a breakthrough arrived.

Was this too good to be true?

"Elementary," said Sherlock Holmes. "It is one of those instances where the reasoner can produce an effect which seems remarkable to his neighbour because the latter has missed the one little point which is the basis of the deduction."[7]

That one "little point" is that hormones derived from natural sources, like plants, have the same basic cell structure as the human body. What is natural, what God has designed, is infinitely better for our bodies than something synthetic, made from the waste matter of pregnant horses.

And now, I invite you, dear reader, to join us on this quest. Please buckle your seat belt and place your trays in the upright position to prepare for landing. Life-changing breakthroughs that have already happened await your attention!

INTRODUCTION

"The Game Is Afoot!"

To quote Sir Arthur Conan Doyle's Sherlock Holmes, "The game is afoot!"[8]

This new medical intervention has already happened, wondrously changing the quality of life for men and women of all ages. It's affordable. It's accessible. The results are profound.

One breakthrough development led to this moment. Leading clinical researchers created and perfected bioidentical pellets for time-release hormone replacement, with minimal side effects, which has proven the best way to restore depleted hormones in the body safely. The Endocrine Society has defined bioidentical hormones as "compounds that have exactly the same chemical and molecular structure as hormones that are produced in the human body."[7]

The biochemical structure is identical to ours. After over nine decades of use (since 1935), it has been shown that bioidentical hormones are the safest and most natural form of hormone replacement. They are created using plant-based ingredients such as yams, soy, and olive oil.

Our bodies recognize this hormone replacement as natural, not foreign. In the past, most hormone replacements were done with synthetic chemicals, many from the urine of pregnant, imprisoned horses. The side effects were worrisome.

Bioidentical hormones are unique because they are, atom for atom, molecule for molecule, and three-dimensionally identical to what our body produces. Therefore, our body recognizes this hormone replacement and reacts positively to this new energy source, unlike anything we have ever experienced. As the small pellets dissolve, they mimic the rate at which natural hormones were released into our bodies when we were young. Their function, metabolism, and elimination are identical to what our body naturally expects. The synthetics are not. The side effects commonly experienced with synthetics have all but disappeared.

Even well-read folks may still need to become familiar with this new option. Most people know a little about hormones and the fact that they have a critical function beyond libido. Then maybe they hear about someone famous who described their life-changing experience of bioidentical hormone replacement in the media.

The first was *New York Times* best-selling author and health guru Suzanne Somers, who has established herself as a leading voice on antiaging. She has written thirteen books on wellness, bioidentical hormones, and how to redefine aging. Suzanne has become a historical figure, a trailblazer, lifting millions of lives by championing the new restoration that awaits us all.

> *I have no bone loss, no brain loss, I have a lot of energy and a lot of strength, my heart is perfect, so I think I'm more ready than I would have been in my 20s, honest to God.*

—SUZANNE SOMERS

We can applaud Ms. Somers for inspiring millions of women to understand the power that hormones can play in their future. Our hormones stimulate the body biochemically. They all work together. Hormones include testosterone, estrogen, progesterone, thyroid hormones, and peptides. Both men and women have this array of hormones that provide energy for the entire body. Over time, hormones dissipate because of age and other reasons. Dramatically.

TIRED OF BEING TIRED

The signs of hormone depletion can begin as early as our twenties. When our hormones begin to fade away, and they are not restored, the problems begin. You may feel exhausted after moderate activity. You may not sleep well. You gain weight and your body aches. You may be cranky. You have brain fog, a fuzzy perception of what's going on. Your alertness has been compromised. Menopause arrives. You may have a vastly reduced libido. Your mind wants to be intimate, but your body does not respond. You are knocking on the door of lousy blood chemistry and type 2 diabetes. Next could be a heart event or a stroke. You may not be motivated to work out or exercise. Perhaps depression knocks on the door. You feel like maybe something has been stolen from you.

LOW HORMONE SYMPTOMS
Men vs Women

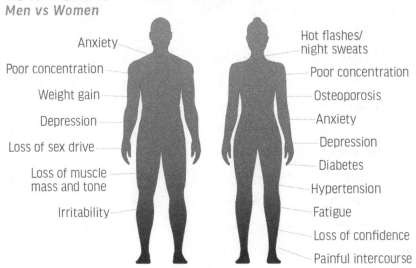

Anxiety
Poor concentration
Weight gain
Depression
Loss of sex drive
Loss of muscle mass and tone
Irritability

Hot flashes/night sweats
Poor concentration
Osteoporosis
Anxiety
Depression
Diabetes
Hypertension
Fatigue
Loss of confidence
Painful intercourse

9

You're frustrated. Here's why: leading researchers suggest that the end-of-life process actually begins with the loss of hormones. It's a downhill run—both for men and for women. Your hormones provide your power source. This "running out of gas" is not a natural aging process.

Everybody's going to age. But what happens if we use the latest technology, the most holistic methods available, to restore the homeostasis balance of our bodies? That is all we're doing. The body itself is brilliant enough to do its work. We're restoring the fuel source without synthetics.

The most common synthetic hormones are unnatural to the human body. Most consist of mixtures of urine from pregnant mares, known as conjugated equine estrogens (CEE) and progestin. All hormones available for therapy are man-made, but synthetic hormones, based on animal cells' structure, can cause bad things to happen in the human body. As *Restore* will show, they can significantly increase your risk of chronic diseases.

This new development of bioidentical time-release hormone replacement pellets represents a breakthrough for men and women. We can now raise hormone levels to your natural, healthy, optimal levels, similar to the structure of your hormones when you were at your peak of youthfulness.

While scientists perfected the formulation of the new hormone pellets, physicians improved the protocols for pellet insertion techniques. In our practice, we worked with colleagues around the country, creating innovations in the insertion process, eliminating almost all the discomfort.

This new pellet dissolves over time, releasing just the right amount of hormones to mimic what our bodies naturally do. Side effects, once common with synthetic hormones, are very minimal. Regular blood tests monitor and demonstrate the impact on your health.

Studies have shown that bioidentical hormone replacement does not increase the chance of having prostate or breast cancer; it makes them less likely.

"Some prescription forms of bioidentical hormones are made by drug companies. The US Food and Drug Administration (FDA) has approved certain bioidentical hormones. Other bioidentical hormones are custom-made by a pharmacist based on a health-care provider's prescription. These are compounded (or mixed) bioidentical hormones," Cleveland Clinic notes.[9]

> **Studies have shown that bioidentical hormone replacement does not increase the chance of having prostate or breast cancer; it makes them less likely.**

Though this new science is not necessarily about increasing our longevity, that could be a result. This is about enjoying robust health for our remaining life span. In other words, our life and health spans become the same.

Science may get even better as time passes, but it has never been this good—ever. In fact, many physicians believe that the widespread use of BHRT will impact the plague of dementia facing our nation.

Sandee LaMotte of *CNN* filed a report on April 5, 2023, suggesting that hormone replacement therapy could be the "sweet spot to avoid dementia."[10]

The *CNN* report noted that Alzheimer's disease strikes women harder than men—over two-thirds of those who descend into dementia's devastating twilight are female at birth. That's likely due to biological reasons that remain poorly understood, according to the Alzheimer's Association.[11]

Gene discovery may explain why more women than men get Alzheimer's disease, LaMotte noted. "A new study may have uncovered a piece or two of the puzzle," she writes. Women who underwent early (age forty to forty-five) or premature (before age forty) menopause, or women who began hormone replacement therapy more than five years after menopause, had higher levels of tau in their brains, according to the study published in the journal *JAMA Neurology*.[12]

Dr. Richard Isaacson, an Alzheimer's preventive neurologist at the Institute for Neurodegenerative Diseases, considered the scientific paper important.[13]

"While it's not the first time a study has shown that early treatment with hormone replacement therapy may be more protective for a woman's brain, it did suggest for the first time that greater amounts of tau protein may be associated with later initiation of hormone treatment," said Isaacson. (Abnormal tau proteins are found in several neurodegenerative diseases.)[14]

Hormone renewal has been provided for many years. It had a rocky period two decades ago. Synthetic hormones caused nasty side effects, and there was fear that they would increase the chances of breast or prostate cancer. The "big reveal" later was that follow-up research showed that these concerns should point only to synthetic hormones.

When I recall my first pellet hormone replacement over a decade ago, I am reminded of the day I first saw an electric Tesla go silently from zero to sixty in less than three seconds. *Wow. This is really true. Time to pay attention to this!*

Do. Not. Blink, I said to myself. *There is something epic going on here.* But now, as you will see in the coming chapters, I will share studies that have confirmed BHRT does not increase the chance of having prostate or breast cancer; it makes them less likely. With these natural bioidentical time-release pellets, all the concerns we experienced with synthetic hormones have vanished.

While new science kept emerging over the next ten years, I did not allow my enthusiasm for these results to get ahead of us. I wrote *The Hormone Handbook* in 2020 as an introduction to BHRT, primarily for my patients. That took off like a rocket, as I explained the full power of this new restoration of the body. For over a decade now, thousands of male and female patients in our practice have enjoyed this restoration with no significant complications.

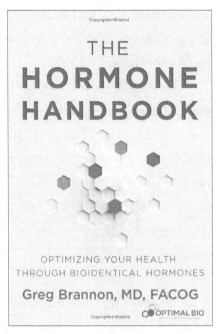

In the coming pages, you will see dozens of clinical studies that conclude that the use of bioidentical hormones can act as a preventative measure and help both men and women improve their health outlook, such as the following:

- Lowers the chance of diabetes

- Improves cognitive ability and mental clarity

- Lowers the risk of Alzheimer's

- Lowers the risk of depression

- Reduces the risk of cancer

- Increases energy levels

- Creates a strong sex drive

- Improves cardiovascular function

- Increases bone density

Restore takes the BHRT discussion to a new level, sharing all the groundbreaking research behind this revolution and interviewing leading researchers, and *Restore* proudly takes us back to the beginning of the human quest for a remedy to the frailties of aging, to the Knights of the Round Table.

We all will grow old. Our bodies will fail. Until the last few years, it seemed a total fantasy to wish for a way to restore our bodies and thus escape the frailty of aging. Yet in the backs of our minds, we felt something was coming from medical science. Something vaguely familiar.

Our culture wishes for this. The excitement about the Holy Grail peaked in recent years when *Indiana Jones and the Last Crusade* dominated box offices worldwide. George Lucas produced the Indiana Jones series as an act of nostalgic affection toward a lost phenomenon. In this film, Indy finds the Holy Grail deep in a mountain. A knight guardian, over seven hundred years old, the last of three brothers who swore an oath to find the grail, guards it. The knight surrenders his sword, pointing Indy and his party to an array of cups of all kinds, advising the seekers:

You must choose.
But choose wisely.
For as the True Grail will bring you life—
The False Grail will take it from you.[15]

The life-changing story we share in this book began over a thousand years ago. We are indeed on a quest to encounter a better way to age well. We all can take part.

It's enjoyable to think back on how we got here. We'll go back briefly to visit the fascinating stories of this worldwide quest to understand the present moment better and observe our forefathers seeking a remedy for the debilitating effects of aging. (Most of these explorers were men, dealing very likely with the same issues facing men today as we experience the growing frailty that comes with age.)

For the first time in history, we have a new choice. We've found the Holy Grail—bioidentical hormone replacement therapy. In *Restore*, I share the human history behind the impulse to seek a remedy for aging and invite you to see the choices you now have and how you can get this beautiful machine God has given us, this beautiful body of ours, back to optimal levels.

Choose wisely. Enjoy the journey!

Chasing the Dream for Centuries

They sought a holy relic, or a fountain of magic water,
to halt aging and reverse the decline all inevitably face.

Restoration of the wellness of the aging human body is a familiar idea. Humanity has been chasing that dream for this past millennium—and more—representing at least forty generations. As far back as the Middle Ages, our ancestors, including the Knights Templar, Ponce de León, and explorers and adventurers throughout the ages, pursued this elusive goal.

Alexander the Great sought a solution as well. The man who conquered most of the known world before he died around 323 BC may have been looking for a river that healed the ravages of age.

Long ago, a medieval king known to Europeans as Prester John supposedly ruled a land with a river of gold and a fountain of youth. Popular stories in Europe in the twelfth to seventeenth centuries depicted Prester John as a descendant of the Three Magi, ruling a kingdom full of riches, marvels, and strange creatures.

Why does there seem to be a bit of nostalgia when we contemplate this? Could the legends passed down over generation after generation of pilgrims be recalled by us on a primal level? Seekers pass along the tales that something out there awaits—just out of reach, getting closer—that can redeem our health and allow us to avoid the inevitable decline. You can say that even today, we have not given up hope.

Scientists and physicians worldwide have been building this new science of *restorative medicine* to halt this decline. As hopeful consumers, we timidly crack the door just enough to peek at recent research, afraid to look too closely, worried we will never be able to afford the cures: the expensive new wonder drug, the six-figure stem cell therapy, the inspirational, charismatic stars promoting cost-prohibitive remedies. As usual, we stand idle, expecting our insurance coverage to not help with the cost.

The solution is now right in front of us. Like in the legends of the Middle Ages and the Knights of the Round Table, now we can act.

It's out there. We're going to find it. It's time to embark upon the age-old quest for youthful wellness in aging. But first, let's go back to where it all began.

DANGEROUS QUESTS

People passed along legends and stories, giving hope to all who would listen. *There may be a way out of this. How shall we follow this dream?* The same drive powered King Arthur and the Knights of the Round Table with visions and rituals to embark upon dangerous quests for the Holy Grail.

Various traditions describe the Holy Grail as a cup, dish, or stone with miraculous healing powers, sometimes providing eternal youth or sustenance in infinite abundance, often guarded in the custody of the Fisher King and located in the hidden grail castle.

By analogy today, folks consider any elusive object or goal of great significance may be perceived as a "Holy Grail" by those seeking a penultimate goal for humanity.

A "grail," wondrous but not unequivocally holy, first appears in *Perceval, the Story of the Grail*, an unfinished chivalric romance written by Chrétien de Troyes around 1190.[16]

Writers portrayed the grail as Jesus's vessel from the Last Supper, which Joseph of Arimathea used to catch Christ's blood at the crucifixion. After that, the Holy Grail became interwoven with the legend of the Holy Chalice, the Last Supper cup, an idea continued in works like the Lancelot-Grail cycle and, consequently, the fifteenth-century *Le Morte d'Arthur*.[17]

For the last five hundred years, this has become a popular theme in modern culture and the subject of pseudohistorical writings and conspiracy theories.

Time marches on. Since then, generations fully believed in the Holy Grail and searched for it, at times frantically racing time to find it. *The cup of a carpenter. The chalice of the son of God*, hidden by a secret sect— somewhere, perhaps with other relics from the crucifixion of Christ.

It became the stuff of Arthurian legend, which many of us read as children. The Knights of the Round Table, Lancelot, and Galahad go on quests to recover the precious cup that would reinvigorate the body and perhaps come with unfathomable powers.

Have I been programmed with instinct? The allure of a quest? A righteous adventure to find a grail? I would like to know if it influenced my decision to become a healer. And my decision to lead my life with a foundation of faith.

The medieval legends of Joseph and Arthur became entwined with the very real and mysterious Knights Templar. This ancient religious order has long been rumored to be the custodians of the grail.

The story of King Arthur and his Knights of the Round Table retells the Arthurian legends. Sir Thomas Malory wrote *Le Morte d'Arthur* in Middle English prose. He told fantastic tales about the legendary King Arthur, Guinevere, Lancelot, Merlin, and the Knights of the Round Table, along with their respective folklore. Lancelot became my favorite, as his swordsmanship and jousting ability gave him all-star status.[18]

But the Knights Templar were not fiction. They were formed in 1120 as a small group of mysterious warrior monks in Jerusalem, headquartered at Solomon's Temple, not far from the tomb of the body of Jesus. They were real.[19]

It sounds like a movie, right?

After the Renaissance, the grail stories fell out of vogue—temporarily. The legend returned to popularity with Richard Wagner's dramatic opera *Parsifal* in 1882, paving the way for a new flood of grail fascination in the modern era, precipitating everything from Nazi rituals to Monty Python, Indiana Jones, and Dan Brown's book and subsequent film *The Da Vinci Code*, which draws heavily from the 1982 book *Holy Blood, Holy Grail*.[20]

For these many years, imaginations lit up, powered by the centuries-long desire to beat nature. Great Britain could just be the place with its castles, knights, monarchs, and stunning landscapes.

For hundreds of years, people have made faithful pilgrimages to the flat Somerset plain; the Glastonbury Tor seems to beckon the pilgrims who journey to this beautiful spot.

Crouched in the lee of three hills, most notably the Tor, the ruins of Glastonbury Abbey are all that remains of "the most significant monastic foundation and church in all of Britain, second only in wealth and size to Westminster." At the height of the Middle Ages, it was a shrine, considered by some as important as Rome itself."[21]

According to legend, this is where Joseph of Arimathea came to reside, the uncle of Jesus who gave up his tomb to house the body of Christ.

Later, the legend goes, "Joseph was given the Holy Grail, the most mystical vessel used to celebrate the Last Supper and the first Eucharist, and which caught some of the blood of the crucified Christ as he hung upon the cross. After the Resurrection, Joseph fled to Britain with the cup and founded the first Christian church on the ancient island of Ynys Witrin, sometimes known as the Glass Isle or Avalon, better known today as Glastonbury."[22]

Long considered the most sacred of the hills, many believe this place to have been the final resting place of the grail.[23]

A spring, rich in iron, which turns the water red, rises here, and a peaceful garden has grown around it in the past decade.[24]

This century alone, there have been sightings of over two hundred different cups[25] throughout Europe. In Asia. In the Caribbean, the South Pacific, and everywhere close to the Holy Land. They're everywhere.

The Chinese, a culture that has practiced disciplined medicine for over five thousand years, had a different approach.[26]

"Feng Geng-sheng, the foremost scholar of traditional Chinese medicines, said the Fountain of Youth—in tablet form—was a secret prescription reserved for Emperor Yongle and his relatives during his Ming Dynasty rule in the 15th century," an article from the *UPI* archives noted.[27]

Of course, a skeptic might point out that Emperor Yongle ruled for twenty-two years after taking power in 1402 but died at sixty-four.

EVILDOERS

Perhaps the evilest human in world history sought the Holy Grail. He wanted to be around for his thousand-year reign. He coveted a painting called the *Ghent Altarpiece*, rumored to contain a coded map to lost Catholic treasures, the so-called Arma Christi, or instruments of Christ's Passion, including the Crown of Thorns, the Holy Grail, and the Spear of Destiny.[28]

Hitler believed that possessing the Arma Christi would grant the owner super-natural powers. As the tide of the war turned ever more against the Nazis, he cranked up his efforts to seek some supernatural way to bring victory to the Third Reich.

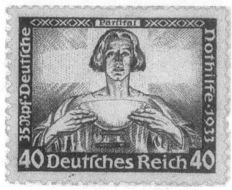

The Holy Grail depicted on a 1933 German stamp

Missions were sent to the Languedoc (in southern France) to find the Holy Grail and to steal the Spear of Destiny, which Longinus used to pierce Christ's side as Christ hung on the cross, which had disappeared from a locked vault in Nurnberg.

Missions also went to Iceland to find the entrance to a magical land called Thule, which Hitler and most of the Nazi brass believed was the place of origin of the Aryans. In the Late Middle Ages and early modern period, the Greco-Roman Thule was often identified with the real Iceland or Greenland.[29]

MAYBE THERE'S ANOTHER WAY: THE FOUNTAIN OF YOUTH

As time passed, wars and the stress of building a nation distracted American people from the Holy Grail quest. There were rumors of it being hidden by the Templars in North America, but not everyone could afford to go on a grail quest. So, inventive as are all Americans, we cheered the finding of the Fountain of Youth, a mythical fountain capable of preserving life that had been fantasized about for centuries.

America did have many hot or warm springs throughout the nation, which we never thought of as a solution to the quest. Long before Europeans landed on the continent, the Native Americans had used the pools routinely for physical therapy and healing. Thomas Jefferson would travel to Warm Springs, Virginia, for weeks to "take the waters."

Jefferson cited the temperature of the warm spring as 96 degrees (Fahrenheit) and that of the hot spring as 112 degrees. He wrote, "They relieve rheumatisms" and that "other complaints also of very different natures have been removed or lessened by them." He noted that the smell would indicate the water to be "sulphureous, as also does the circumstance of its turning silver black."[30]

With thousands of soldiers recovering from the hideous Civil War, exuberant entrepreneurs created a magical place to heal and restore youthful wellness, and not just any fountain would do. This was *the* Fountain of Youth.

The name linked most closely to this search is sixteenth-century Spanish explorer Juan Ponce de León, who allegedly thought it would be found in Florida. In Saint Augustine, the oldest city in the United States, there's a tourist attraction dating back over a century that purports—albeit tongue in cheek—to be the Fountain of Youth.

Saint Augustine, Florida, celebrates this site, where "Ponce de León first set foot in America." *Maybe so. Maybe not.*

But the appealing tale of the search for a Fountain of Youth survives anyway, says Ryan K. Smith, a professor of history at Virginia Commonwealth University, commenting in a recent *New York Times* article on the nature of the mystery.

"People are more intrigued by the story of looking and not finding than they are by the idea that the fountain might be out there somewhere,"[31] Smith says.

"Juan Ponce de León was obsessed with the Fountain of Youth, the story goes. This obsession led him to discover Florida, through whose impossible jungles he drove his men on suicide missions. Bugs, bears, alligators, snakes, sinkholes, natives: Nothing could stop Ponce. He was the Spanish inland Ahab. He had to have his sip of the magic water. What's a suicide mission if it leads to eternal life?"[32]

Ponce de León, of course, never found the Fountain of Youth. He'd still be here to tell us about it if he had. Instead, he died. In 1521, on the Gulf Coast, he was shot in the thigh with an arrowhead carved out of a fishbone.[33]

Ponce de León had sailed to the Americas with Christopher Columbus. He knew how costly these journeys were and all the possible ways they could go wrong. He sailed to Florida in search of the usual colonial obsessions: land, gold, and enslaved people.

Thus, we made him a hero and the historical founder of Florida. *Whoops.*

The *New York Times* reminds us, "Elderly visitors who drink the spring's sulfur-smelling water don't turn into teenagers."[34]

Luella Day McConnell created the tourist attraction in its present form in 1904. Having abandoned her practice as a physician in Chicago and gone to the Yukon during the Klondike gold rush of the 1890s, she purchased the park property with cash and diamonds. She became known in Saint Augustine as "Diamond Lil," a nickname people gave her while she chased gold in Alaska.[35]

Around 1909, she began advertising the attraction, charging admission, and selling postcards and water from a well dug in 1875. A cup of the healing water cost ten cents. But wait. There's more. Today's bargain rates are for adults: $19.95; seniors: $17.95; children six to twelve: $9.95; children five and under: free. Special rates are available for Saint Johns County Residents and tour groups of ten or more.

As we gracefully make the turn from wishing about rejuvenation to being quite able to enjoy it, there's another dimension to this desire. It does seem a bit nostalgic. As you can see, seeking youthful wellness in aging has been ingrained in our culture, perhaps in our DNA, since the Middle Ages. It's all so familiar for some reason. It's like a baby that takes swimming lessons before age one, born with the basic knowledge and ability to swim.

The search for the answer to frailty in aging moved from expeditions on horseback to clinical laboratories all over the world.

Now that we have legitimate choices today, we have a significant advantage over the Grail seekers and the Fountain of Youth devotees, who bumped from place to place, perhaps frantically hoping to get lucky.

Our scientists do not rely on luck or legend. The big difference now in this era is that the search for the answer to frailty in aging moved from expeditions on horseback to clinical laboratories all over the world. The speed with which medical advancements have occurred during this century is staggering.

This vast knowledge in medical science has been steadily marching forward, forcing our best and brightest physicians to specialize, to focus on one disease, one aspect of health, or one body system. The pace of advancements lends weight to the idea that, yes, a remedy for the frailty of aging nears. In our lifetime, hormone replacement, stem cell research, and miracle drugs are all on the table for many of us. For some, it's too early to choose. For hormone replenishment, the time has arrived. You must choose. For some of these advancing technologies, the choice is not yet here. For hormone restoration, choose wisely!

Indy rushes forward and pushes Donovan away. As he falls, his body breaks into flames, then shatters against the wall.

Grail Knight. He chose … poorly.

Indy studies the array of chalices.

Elsa. It would not be made out of gold.

Indy picks up another cup,
a simple earthenware jug.

Indy. That's the cup of a carpenter.

He and Elsa exchange a look.

Indy. There's only one way to find out.[36]

2

Pinch Yourself— You May Now Restore Your Body Chemistry

I've always wanted to be a crusader, like the Knights of the Round Table, who rode off on missions to protect the pilgrims traveling to the Holy Land. I wanted to be like them—a noble knight, protecting what's right, serving a higher calling. I wanted my talent and passion to mean something.

Restoring your optimal hormone level has become easy, affordable, and accessible. This will lay the cornerstone for a different life than you are experiencing now. It solves the problems we just listed. Through the power of bioidentical hormones, energy flows back into your body. It helps your intestinal tract, your heart, your bones, the prostate, the breasts, your relationships, your mood, and your outlook. It helps every cell.

The optimal health of our cells peaks when we are eighteen to twenty-six years old. *Remember those days?* All systems go. All our hormones were at "optimal" levels. Full tank. Flash forward a few decades later, and everything changes. But it does not have to be that way.

You cannot drive a combustion car without oxygen. Oxygen combusts with gasoline. There's your explosion. The car, the fluid, and the actual gas symbolize our testosterone, primarily estrogen, progesterone, and the thyroid, the T3 and reverse T3 ratio; that's the combustion.

A recent seventy-two-year-old male patient said this about five weeks after receiving the pellet insertion: "I've felt like this before, something I welcome back," he said. "I felt like this when I was twenty-five years old."

We call the result "graceful aging," and I was present at its birth. In ten years, we have done hormone replacement with bioidentical hormones for thousands of men and women without any severe side effects. Based on my own experience and the data I've gathered through the years, over 98 percent of our patients are thrilled with their optimal hormone levels. In addition, we have fine-tuned the process, making it much more accessible, entirely natural, and quicker than ten years ago.

BENEFITS FOR WOMEN

Bioidentical hormone replacement can treat and improve a broad spectrum of problems in women, including weight gain, brain fog, low energy, insomnia, low libido, adrenal fatigue, MS, memory loss, and migraines. Vast improvement occurs for other problems, such as chronic fatigue syndrome, post-traumatic stress disorder, depression, autoimmune disease, hypothyroidism, and metabolic syndrome. Muscle tone improves. Libido improves. You feel young again.

If suffering from menopause or perimenopause, women experience immediate and lifelong relief. It also restores women who have had a full or partial hysterectomy.

Undo the Harm

In the spring of 2021, a prominent scientist who doubted hormone therapy the most decades earlier recanted his criticism. "Today, USC medical researcher Howard Hodis, MD, is driven by a singular goal: to prove the benefits of hormone replacement therapy and undo the harm he says has been done to women's health over the past twenty years. He runs a multimillion-dollar, National Institutes of Health-funded study to see how hormone replacement therapy affects women's thinking and cardiovascular health," observed USC writer Katherine Gammon.[37]

"Hormone replacement therapy is linked to cutting the number one cause of death by about half for the women who opted to take it," said Dr. Hodis, who holds the Harry J. Bauer and Dorothy Bauer Rawlins Professorship in Cardiology at the Keck School of Medicine of USC.[38]

His new mission was vividly described in an article by Katherine Gammond in the Spring 2021 USC website entitled "It's Time to Rethink Hormone Therapy for Women, Says Heart Health Scientist."[39]

"That has implications for quality of life and longevity, given that 53 percent of US women die from cardiovascular disease. Hormone therapy also helps prevent bone loss, which is critical for older women. One in ten women who break their hip after age 70 die," Gammond noted.[40]

"Hormone replacement therapy contains the female hormone estrogen, restoring some women's estrogen levels that decline as they age. Besides fighting hot flashes, it helps prevent bone loss and fractures. Over twenty years, though, large studies observing women's health also noticed something else: Those on the therapy had less heart disease, the leading killer of American women," Gammon explained.[41]

Cardiovascular Disease:
The Number-One Killer of Women

Howard N. Hodis, MD and Wendy J. Mack, PhD, of the Keck School of Medicine, University of Southern California, reminded us in an article published in 2022, that cardiovascular disease causes 1 in 3.2 deaths in women each year in the United States, noting that cardiovascular disease (CVD) remains the number one killer of women, accounting for approximately one death every eighty seconds.[42]

Their study noted that eye-opening differences exist between women and men in presentation, outcomes and pathophysiological mechanisms making CVD a more severe disease for women than men.[43]

- For example, 64 percent of women versus 50 percent of men who die suddenly of coronary heart disease (CHD) have no previous symptoms.

- In addition, more women than men die within one year (23 percent of women versus 18 percent of men) (and within five years 47 percent of women versus 36 percent of men) after a first myocardial infarction (MI).

- More women than men develop heart failure (22 percent of women versus 16 percent of men) and suffer a stroke (7 percent of women versus 4 percent of men) within five years of a first MI.

- Further, more women than men have a recurrent MI or fatal CHD (21 percent of women versus 17 percent of men) within five years after a first MI.[44]

The authors concluded that when hormone replacement therapy is initiated in women less than sixty years of age and/or at or near menopause, "HRT significantly reduces all-cause mortality and cardiovascular disease (CVD) whereas other primary CVD prevention therapies such as lipid-lowering fail to do so. Magnitude and type of HRT-associated risks, including breast cancer, stroke, and venous thromboembolism are rare (less than 10 events per 10,000 women), not unique to HRT and comparable with other medications. HRT is a sex-specific and time-dependent primary CVD prevention therapy that concomitantly reduces all-cause mortality as well as other aging-related diseases with an excellent risk profile."[45]

Women Have Been Misled about Menopause[46]

New York Times reporter Susan Dominus published an article on February 1, 2023, highlighting the "overlooked" remedies for most of the symptoms of menopause:

> Hot flashes, sleeplessness, pain during sex: For some of menopause's worst symptoms, there's an established treatment. Why aren't more women offered it?
>
> Now imagine that there was a treatment for all these symptoms that doctors often overlooked. The scenario seems unlikely, yet it's a depressingly accurate picture of menopausal care for women. There is a treatment, hardly obscure, known as menopausal hormone therapy, that eases hot flashes and sleep disruption, and possibly depression and aching joints. It decreases the risk of diabetes and protects against osteoporosis. It also helps prevent and treat menopausal genitourinary syndrome, a collection of symptoms, including urinary tract infections and pain during sex, that affects nearly half of postmenopausal women.[47]

Hormone treatment has been proven to increase bone density significantly. But it matters what type of hormone treatment you use. The *American Journal of Obstetrics and Gynecology* has demonstrated a fourfold increase in bone density with bioidentical hormones over oral estrogen and a two-and-a-half times greater increase in bone density than with hormone patches. The details of those increases for women are as follows:

- A 1–2 percent increase in bone density per year with oral estrogen

- A 3.5 percent increase in bone density per year with patches

- An 8.3 percent increase in bone density per year with pellet therapy[48]

BENEFITS FOR MEN

"Testosterone can be your silver bullet," says author Jay Campbell in his 2015 book *The Definitive Testosterone Replacement Therapy Manual.*

"The science of this is indisputable," Campbell notes. "Testosterone, when administered properly and in clinical dose fashion, has the potential to revitalize male life across every conceivable aspect of health, whether musculature, improved metabolic health, or improved cognitive and psychologic benefits."[49]

Harvard urologist and author of a landmark book that made all this possible, Dr. Abraham Morgantaler, noted in a 2021 article in *Life Extension Magazine* that in men, there's "a persistent fear of prostate cancer and the belief that T therapy causes the disease continues to influence physicians and patients alike."[50] But for decades, Morgentaler and other scientists aggressively challenged that assumption.

"Long-term studies looking for increased incidence of prostate cancer in men with naturally high T levels have consistently failed to show any relationship at all," notes Dr. Morgentaler.[51]

"Other studies showed that PSA was unchanged in men who received treatment that increased their T levels to more than twice the 'normal' range." Dr. Morgentaler has published data showing that men with significant *reductions in testosterone levels* have an increased risk for prostate cancer!"[52]

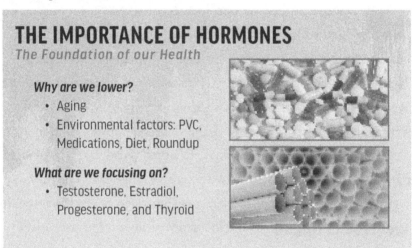

THE IMPORTANCE OF HORMONES
The Foundation of our Health

Why are we lower?
- Aging
- Environmental factors: PVC, Medications, Diet, Roundup

What are we focusing on?
- Testosterone, Estradiol, Progesterone, and Thyroid

Other world-class researchers became interested. A "pooled data" study by dozens of scientists in the Endogenous Hormones, Prostate Cancer Collaborative Group and published in the *Journal of the National Cancer Institute* reviewed prospective studies that included 3,886 men with prostate cancer and 6,438 control subjects. The studies evaluated the risk of prostate cancer, total and free testosterone levels, and other sex hormones. The conclusion?

"In this collaborative analysis of the worldwide data on endogenous hormones and prostate cancer risk, serum concentrations of sex hormones were not associated with the risk of prostate cancer."[53]

A SEVEN-YEAR STUDY OF OVER FOUR HUNDRED THOUSAND PATIENTS

Researcher and OB/GYN physician Gary S. Donovitz, MD, FACOG, FRSM, recently published "A Personal Perspective on Testosterone Therapy in Women—What We Know in 2022" in the *Journal of Personalized Medicine.*

Dr. Donovitz calls attention to a recent seven-year retrospective study that looked back at 1.2 million subcutaneous hormone-pellet implant procedures performed in four hundred thousand patients. The overall continuation after two insertions was 93 percent, and the overall complication rate was less than 1 percent.[54]

> **I've seen lives change. Every day patients tell us we have changed their lives ... every single day.**

"The study demonstrated long-term safety,"[55] he noted. In addition, he pointed to two extensive long-term peer-reviewed studies showing a significant reduction in the incidence of invasive breast cancer in women on testosterone therapy.[56]

"Perhaps it is time for the FDA to consider approving products that would benefit testosterone-deficient women," he concluded.[57]

As an ob-gyn, I can confidently say there are no words to express the physician's joy in helping parents deliver their babies. Yet now that my wife, Jody, and I are experiencing this rejuvenation, we share our patients' enthusiasm as they regain their youthfulness daily. I am jubilant, a joy similar to my decades of easing new life into the world.

I've seen lives change. Every day patients tell us we have changed their lives ... every single day.

I have enjoyed my patients returning for their checkups, grinning from ear to ear. Name another branch of medicine that nearly every patient returns to you thrilled with the results. Now you know why—after the first few years of offering this science to my patients, I stopped everything and reluctantly ceased my practice of OB/GYN to perfect pellet insertion techniques and master dosage algorithms to help bring this innovation to our culture. I could not get over the fact that almost every patient was thrilled with the therapy. I thought the response would be excellent, but almost everybody? That's pretty rare in medicine.

People are choosing well to make their remaining years full of vitality and energy.

A sense of destiny comes with my work now. An inner excitement that I have been present at the birth of something wondrous. I urge you to embrace this most excellent opportunity in our lifetime to begin aging gracefully.

"There are less obvious reasons to be concerned about declining testosterone levels—reasons that relate to total body health, not just behavior and performance, sexual or otherwise, according to Canadian expert Dr. Jerald Bain.[58]

"Testosterone is more than a 'male sex hormone.' It is an important contributor to the robust metabolic functioning of multiple bodily systems."

Harvard urologist and pioneer of testosterone therapy Dr. Abraham Morgentaler concurs vehemently.

"Testosterone stimulates and maintains muscle and bone growth, for example—many men don't realize that low T puts them at increased risk for osteoporosis with advancing age. It also stimulates red blood cell production, helping to prevent anemia."[59]

Testosterone levels are reduced in type 2 diabetes and metabolic syndrome. Although the cause and effect remain unclear, therapy with testosterone in these conditions can reduce LDL cholesterol, blood sugar, glycated hemoglobin, and insulin resistance.

Finally, Dr. Morgentaler notes, "Men with low T die earlier than those with normal T."[60]

"That alone is ample reason to take notice," Dr. Morgantaler explains.[61]

When asked, "Why should we care?" Dr. Morgentaler replied, "If I told you of a known medication that can improve mood and performance while reducing the risks for a host of chronic, apparently age-related conditions and has the real potential for increasing longevity, you would jump at it. There's solid evidence for all of that with responsible testosterone replacement therapy. Men who feel old, have decreased 'get up and go,' and diminished sex drive may not simply be 'getting old;' they may be suffering from a treatable hormone deficiency."[62]

In his book *Ageless, The New Science of Getting Older Without Getting Old*, Dr. Andrew Steele discusses how "Aging—not cancer, not heart disease—is the underlying cause of most human death and suffering. The same cascade of biological changes that renders us wrinkled and gray also opens the door to dementia and disease. We work furiously to conquer each individual disease, but we never think to ask: Is aging itself necessary?"[63]

After earning a PhD in physics from the University of Oxford, Andrew Steele decided that aging was the single most important scientific challenge of our time and switched fields to computational biology.

He notes, "Nature tells us that are tortoises and salamanders who are spry into old age and whose risk of dying is the same no matter how old they are, a phenomenon known as 'biological immortality.'"

In *Ageless*, Andrew Steele charts the astounding progress science has made in recent years to secure the same for humans: to help us become old without getting frail, to live longer without ill health or disease."[64]

The Guardian writer Alex Moshakis tells the story of Andrew Steele's experiences when he says to people that we might one day cure aging as if it were any other disease: "They are often incredulous and sometimes hostile. Once, at a friend's wedding, he left a group of guests mildly incensed for suggesting that near-future humans might live well into their 100s. A similar thing happens at dinner parties, where the responses are more polite but no less skeptical. He understands the reaction. We think of aging as an inescapable fact of life—we're born, we grow old, so it goes. 'That's been the narrative for thousands of years,'" he says. 'But what if it didn't have to be?'"[65]

I wonder what the families of the Crusaders thought as their beloved knights rode off into the wilderness to protect pilgrims or search for the Holy Grail. What if they found it? What would they do? When would they return from the quest? What if enemies outnumbered them?

I am sure there were skeptics then as they watched the riders disappear into the unknown over the horizon.

In the last decade, we have seen the same human sentiments arise when this magnificent scientific breakthrough was first brought forward. Many people could not comprehend the global significance of this bioidentical hormone replacement and the powerful impact it could have on our lives. Folks could understand that our hormones diminish over time as we age, but that's where the belief paused, as we waited for evidence, as we waited for more people to cheer the result.

The magnificent work of the researchers and scientists had to wait a bit. They held onto their upper-atmosphere ambitions and kept moving forward.

This was not a pill, the usual form of response to an illness or pain. Folks had never known that their hormones were diminishing as they aged, and even more to the point, few knew that a solid answer was emerging. Pills do not work as well as a carefully inserted, dissolving, all-natural pellet for this therapy. Pills must pass all the way through the digestive system, and their impact would be significantly lessened and create unwanted side effects along the way.

So the pioneers calmly kept up their pace, grappling with the doubt, continuing their quest because it is important to everybody. They were keeping their eyes on the North Star.

Imagine, for the first time in medical history,
being able to miraculously change the way we age.

Healthcare around the world changes in steady incremental steps. Even the best breakthroughs must slowly integrate into what we do as a culture. First, you need indisputable success. Then you need a body of believers. So here we are. There are now millions of believers. The awakening has begun.

I think that adolescent vision led me to become a doctor. I even envisioned my mom sending me out on a quest one day. Well, she did, and off I went to become a doctor, and I was trained at USC (at what had to be one of the best schools in the world for OB/GYN). My mentors wrote the textbooks on obstetrics and gynecology.

If you had asked me twenty-five years ago, I would never have foreseen my medical career move into wellness and graceful aging. I got my start in learning about prevention. But flash forward a quarter of a century, and the crusader in me would awaken. Again.

While I loved OB/GYN, and especially helping a new life into this world, I was attracted to prevention as the part of functional health that I believe represents the cornerstone, the foundation, of future healthcare. That's very important to understand. I was about to live this myself.

My journey took me through delivering thousands of babies and the pure joy of working with moms. Jody and I have seven wonderful children.

I began to evolve in how I approached medicine. My crusade at the time was in breaking the mold of current medical practice that has abandoned the Marcus Welby home-visit mentality.

As an OB/GYN practice, I had a marvelous staff who embraced the idea that when we meet every patient, they should instantly know we care about them as individuals. I have always felt deeply that practicing medicine any other way is missing the point.

We did home visits for urgent breastfeeding issues, fevers, or post-surgical pain. Here's an example of how we did things in my practice:

I got a phone call from a patient; let's call her Jeanne. Something was not right with her breastfeeding. She was scared. This is not a situation where I would phone in a drug. On this day, I asked my wife, Jody, to accompany me as a chaperone (always advised), and off we went to her home. I examined her and suggested that she apply heat to her breasts and keep pressing and said she would be fine. I could see the relief on her face when I walked in the door. She was better the next day.

I would arrive at her house when patients indicated they were afraid or frantic. We did that for years. As I got busier, I brought a labor nurse on board, who would help me with the home visits. We would never charge for it.

In medicine, the unknown is the scariest.

No need for you to come in. I'll be right over.

If a patient discovers a breast lump, I'll see her that day. Forget about being busy. If a patient is bleeding, it's urgent that I get there. Yeast infections hurt. *Let's go.* There is great truth in the healer's touch.

Showing up is half the cure. I was delivering eighty babies a month, but I was seeing my patients when they needed me. That's what motivated me. That's why I became a doctor. To be a trusted healer.

A trusted healer shows up. *Perhaps a knight. Perhaps in shining armor. Well, I can still tap into all that when I want to.*

So you can see why giving up this spiritually fulfilling practice might have been impossible.

But I found myself running to a new development in medicine. One that would change the lives of my patients and help nudge the entire world into a new way of aging. And that would make me the crusader I always wanted to be.

I did not know what awaited me in my personal health or the breakthrough that would cure me of a chronic disease—a severe kidney infection. I was marching briskly on the road to full-blown diabetes and could see the barn ahead. For an unknown reason, I experienced severe inflammation of my kidneys. My body was under attack. I had to start taking care of myself.

My wife, Jody, and I started reading all the latest literature and studying the phenomenon I experienced. I attacked my silent enemy's approach to diabetes. For type 1 diabetes, physicians must give insulin, which makes sense because your pancreas is not making insulin.

For type 2 diabetes, which I was currently enduring, our bodies make insulin, but the receptor is resistant, so our physicians give us more.

So we inquired. What if we attacked sugar, a major aggravating substance?

We've always been told to abide by the food pyramid that we learned in school, which quite frankly has become the absolute worst diet we could possibly have. Almost the whole country is obese and dealing with chronic diseases now because of that. The issue of *truth* lit up like a Christmas tree. Who's telling us this?

As a culture, we keep doing what we're told is good.

Here are the facts: I had a chronic illness, and looking back, I was abiding by the good old food pyramid we learned in school, which, quite frankly, did some real harm to my body. *Here's how we eat!* Our nation embraced this as the best dietary practice.

> *Over the past one hundred years, our species has been engaged in a vast and complicated chemistry experiment. Every one of us, along with our children, our parents, and our grandparents, has been a guinea pig in this experiment, which uses our bodies, our health, and our goodwill to test the proposition that modern science can improve upon the foods and medicines of nature.*
>
> —RANDALL FITZGERALD, *THE HUNDRED-YEAR LIE: HOW FOOD AND MEDICINE ARE DESTROYING YOUR HEALTH*

Jody and I asked ourselves the question, *How did we get here?* We knew the original intention was to create something other than the culture of terrible health habits and diet we currently navigate. As in so many ways, our population has served as the guinea pig for many ventures in health, and we're seeing the results of it now. The food pyramid champions were dead wrong.

Here's the elephant in the room: *we may free ourselves from doing everything we're told.*

Finally, Jody and I created a three-part plan to save me from diabetes. My cure, which is still ongoing, had three parts. I had to lose weight and get in better shape. I was a weight-trained triathlete, and that was the good part. But I had to lose weight and get the sugar out of my diet. And my insulin crisis had taken a toll on my hormones. I needed hormone replacement therapy.

So you can see why I did not run from this spiritually fulfilling medical practice; I ran to a thrilling new development in medicine.

REMEMBERING AN ICON IN MEDICINE: DANIEL R. MISHELL JR., MD

When the flawed Women's Health Initiative study came out in 2002 (which I describe in detail shortly), unnecessarily scaring the medical establishment about the risks of hormone replacement, I called my mentor, Dr. Dan Mishell (1936–2016) at USC, where I served my residency.

Dr. Mishell wrote most of the most reputable books on menopause, obstetrics, and gynecology; his legacy is everlasting.

Dr. Mishell spent most of his career in the Department of Obstetrics and Gynecology at the Keck School of Medicine of USC, which I view as one of the top residency programs in the nation. He led the department for over forty years, serving as chairman, research mentor, and friend—always generously sharing his clinical insights, intellectual acumen, and passion for women's health.

I asked Dr. Mishell (I always called him that!), "How can these people totally ignore positive clinical research, ignoring over seventy-seven years of positive research citing the benefits of hormone replacement? From 1935 to 2002, virtually every single paper said hormones were beneficial until this one paper came out ... how do you throw seventy-years years of literature out the door?"

He replied, "Greg, I trained you well. Never give up."

That conversation got me thinking about BHRT, and I never looked back. We've been fighting this rabbit hole of falsehoods for years.

I owe a debt of gratitude to an OB/GYN colleague in Scottsdale, Arizona—Gino Tutero, MD, who pioneered the use of bioidentical pellets for hormonal replacement. I went to a conference he held in Arizona, and for three days, I argued with him. And for three days, he refuted every scientific argument I could throw at him. He convinced me that this was an advancement of global significance. It was a powerful experience, and I was all in.

I came home, did the pellet replacement therapy on myself with the assistance of my physician assistant, and I opened a bioidentical hormone replacement facility near my OB/GYN office the next day.

A few weeks passed. The reaction in my body was not immediate. Then, a couple of weeks following the placement of bioidentical hormone pellets, it was like watching a slowly clearing sky reveal a full moon behind thin clouds. I was not expecting the rush of mental clarity, but it was terrific. My energy came out of hiding. My body felt better. *This is an adventure that keeps getting better and better every day.*

I realized something epic was taking place. *It felt like summer lightning … surprising, awe-inspiring—beautiful.*

That's how this advancement hit me. I would never offer a new clinical advancement to my family or patients until I tried it myself. After a few weeks, seeing the impact on me, Jody asked me to have my physician assistant perform her hormone replacement, hoping to resolve some symptoms she was experiencing. I told her to *brace herself for something you have not felt in a long time.* Weeks later, we both felt immensely better.

"Where has this been?" she asked.

A few weeks later, Jody and I compared notes with energy. We were becoming acquainted with the incredible results of this fantastic new therapy.

One morning, we were getting ready for our day. She touched my hand, something she does when she needs to break me out of my reclusive mental pace. She got my attention.

We both feel … entirely different. So … where's this been my whole life?

She looks twenty years younger. Her energy level, mental acuity, mood, and muscular toning all transformed. Her tiredness diminished, despite caring for seven kids. Her mind is sharp as a whip. Earlier, she stopped using synthetic hormones; now, the full results emerged six weeks into the bioidentical therapy. I thought about what she said for a moment.

Soon, my extra weight disappeared, my muscle tone vastly improved, my hyperalertness kicked in (I've been told I drive people crazy), and my blood numbers improved.

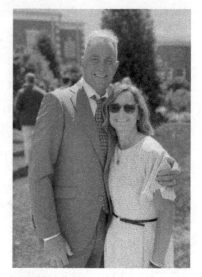

I replied to Jody, "They told us wrong, that's what. Where's this been? It's been here all along."

I asked Jody to share her experience with us.

Dr. Greg Brannon and his wife, Jody

Jody's Story

"One day, I was driving around town with my daughter in tow, and I suddenly had no idea where I was or where I was going. Could I possibly be experiencing early onset memory loss? I was only in my forties. I was also experiencing fatigue and muscle loss and had trouble sleeping. I chalked it all up to aging, motherhood, and running a busy household. As time went on, symptoms continued to get worse. I can age gracefully, but would I have to be in such discomfort in so many areas of my life?

"My husband, Greg, was beginning to talk about hormone replacement pellets. I listened, but I am naturally a skeptic and a bit of a chicken when it comes to medical intervention. But one day, I decided to 'bite the bullet.' Within days, my memory fog was easing up, and my sleep patterns began to regulate. My biggest surprise was the physical changes ... muscle tone, hair texture, and tightening of my skin. Again, I am happy to grow old gracefully, but I am so excited to age with health and energy and be able to experience new adventures along the way."

Why are we not embracing the holistic replenishment of our body's diminished hormones, which affect every organ? Know that bioidentical restorative therapy represents a cultural breakthrough. Men and women of all ages can benefit. What if we restored the hormones of every American adult who chooses to renew their energy sources? Decades ago, the FDA approved synthetic therapies, complete with the side effects that come when man tries to outwit nature. We have something much better now.

An excellent example is that our medical establishment did not ignore diabetes; they discovered how to replace the lost insulin for the patient's survival. At first, they used farm animals for synthetic insulin. But we were grateful for the discovery. Lives were saved. But there were some side effects and the increased threat of chronic disease. Vastly superior bioidentical insulin replaced synthetic insulin years ago. That's wonderful, but why have we not adopted bioidentical hormones as the default hormone replacement? *What's up with that?* Synthetic hormones, synthetically made from urine from pregnant mares, can cause some troublesome side effects.

I feel a crusade coming on.

So do not be shocked. This quest has been going on for centuries. But think about this: science has exploded in the last fifty years. We have landed humans on the moon. Our scientists have invented antibiotics, digital medical records, robotic surgery, and artificial intelligence, halted major plagues, and now, we have opened the door to graceful aging. We have finally arrived at a cultural moment of contemplation. We have not found everlasting life duration on the planet, but we have found something that will make the ride to the end much more pleasant.

I love being here. I loved my choice to champion this breakthrough over ten years ago. I love the advancements we have made in bioidentical hormones—clinical body chemistry monitoring, pellet placement, and long-term effects. I have stared down skeptics by asking, *What is wrong with attacking the aging process with all the science we can muster?*

My colleagues and I have pushed back against the medical-industrial complex, reminding me of the resistance the Crusaders provided in fending off the brutal enemies of the pilgrimage. Defending the truth brings welcome companions.

We have deflected a skeptical bureaucracy that hasn't gotten much right since we have ceded medicine to this unholy alliance of bloated insurance companies and government medical overreach. The knights are coming home victorious; the delicate twinkling of their armor can be seen on the horizon. Mission accomplished. The Eagle has landed.

Pinch yourself.

My mentor, Dr. Dan Mishell, was absolutely right when he gave me my professional mantra, "Never give up." And I never looked back.

We've been fighting this rabbit hole of falsehoods for years. Here's a great synopsis on this clinical revolution published in 2019 by Angelo Cagnacci and Martina Venier entitled "The Controversial History of Hormone Replacement Therapy."

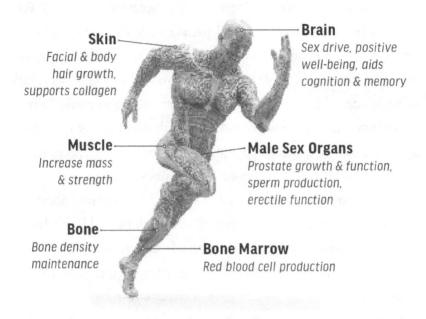

Skin
Facial & body
hair growth,
supports collagen

Brain
Sex drive, positive
well-being, aids
cognition & memory

Muscle
Increase mass
& strength

Male Sex Organs
Prostate growth & function,
sperm production,
erectile function

Bone
Bone density
maintenance

Bone Marrow
Red blood cell production

Just a few roles of testosterone in the body

THE CONTROVERSIAL HISTORY OF HORMONE REPLACEMENT THERAPY

A re-analysis of the Women's Health Initiative (WHI) trial was performed, and new studies showed that the use of BHRT in younger women or early postmenopausal women had a beneficial effect on the cardiovascular system, reducing coronary disease and all-cause mortality. Notwithstanding, public opinion on HRT has not changed yet, leading to important negative consequences for women's health and quality of life.[66]

September 2019

The controversial history of Hormone Replacement Therapy (HRT) is about the history of a powerful pathogenetic therapy for all post-menopausal disturbances. Its effects on symptoms are and were immediately visible, at first prompting rapidly growing estrogen use. A lack of knowledge about its side effects and complications, particularly in the endometrium, prompted consequences that limited HRT use. Subsequent association with progestin allowed for the widespread use of HRT, with favorable consequences on many aspects of women's health.

Unfortunately, the surge in HRT use and its consolidation was abruptly stopped by the publication of the Women's Health Initiative (WHI) trial, which was inadequately designed, evaluated, and reported. The damage was huge, leaving many symptomatic women without an effective treatment, even if the epidemiological data were not strong enough to document a clear harm to women's health. Although most of the evidence obtained was only with oral conjugated estrogen with or without medroxyprogesterone acetate, further studies and analyses have consolidated the view that HRT is highly beneficial when given to symptomatic women within ten years since the onset of menopause or to symptomatic women that are under 60 years of age. However, the damage remains, and low HRT use, which is unjustified, continues to occur worldwide.[67]

I have included the references for a critical clinical analysis on the next page to magnify the scientific community's intense focus on this topic in recent years. I invite you to visit some of these groundbreaking studies to note the intense worldwide support for hormone replacement.

REFERENCES

"The Controversial History of Hormone Replacement Therapy"
Angelo Cagnacci and Martina Venier
September 18, 2019

The authors of this study provide this reference list, which gives us a glimpse of the vast knowledge and scientific study that has led up to the bioidentical hormone replacement therapy advancements worldwide.

1. Keep P.A., Kellerhals J. The ageing woman. In: Lauritzen C., van Keep P.A., editors. Ageing and Estrogens. Frontiers of Hormone Research, **Proceedings of the 1st International Workshop on Estrogen Therapy**, Geneva, Switzerland, 1972. Volume 2. S. Karger; Basel, Switzerland: 1973. pp. 160–173.

2. Kling J. **The Strange Case of Premarin Modern Drug Discovery**. [(accessed [CrossRef] [Google Scholar] on 22 July 2019)];2000 Available online: http://pubs.acs.org/subscribe/archive/mdd/v03/i08/html/kling.html

3. Wilson R.A. In: In **Feminine Forever.** Evans M., editor. Lippincott & Co.; Philadelphia, PA, USA: 1996.

4. Ziel H.K., Finkle W.D. **Increased risk of endometrial carcinoma among users of conjugated estrogens**. N. Engl. J. Med. 1975293:1167–1170. doi: 10.1056/NEJM197512042932303.

5. Smith D.C., Prentice R., Thomson D.J., Herrmann W.L. **Association of exogenous estrogen and endogenous carcinoma.** N. Engl. J. Med. 1975293:1164–1167. doi: 10.1056/NEJM197512042932302. [PubMed] [CrossRef] [Google Scholar]

6. Woodruff J.D., Pickar J.H. **Incidence of endometrial hyperplasia in postmenopausal women taking conjugated estrogens (Premarin) with medroxyprogesterone acetate or conjugated estrogens alone.** The Menopause Study Group. Am. J. Obstet. Gynecol. 1994170:1213–1223. doi: 10.1016/S0002-9378(13)90437-3.

7. Lobo R.A. **Hormone-replacement therapy: Current thinking.** Nat. Rev. Endocrinol. 2017;1 220–231. doi: 10.1038/nrendo.2016.164.

8. North American Menopause Society **The 2012 hormone therapy position statement of the North American Menopause Society.** Menopause. 2012;19: 257–271. doi: 10.1097/ gme.0b013e31824b970a. [PMC free article] [

9. Grodstein F., Stampfer M.J., Colditz G.A., Willett W.C., Manson J.E., Joffe M., Rosner B., Fuchs C., Hankinson S.E., Hunter D.J., et al. **Postmenopausal hormone therapy and mortality.** N. Engl. J. Med. 1997;336: 1769–1775. doi: 10.1056/ NEJM199706193362501

10. Yaffe K., Sawaya G., Lieberburg I., Grady D. **Estrogen therapy in postmenopausal women: Effects on cognitive function and dementia.** JAMA. 1998;279: 688–695. doi: 10.1001/ jama.279.9.688.

11. Stampfer M.J., Colditz G.A. **Estrogen replacement therapy and coronary heart disease: A quantitative assessment of the epidemiologic evidence.** Prev. Med. 1991;20: 47–63. doi: 10.1016/0091-7435(91)90006-P.

12. Grady D., Rubin S.M., Petitti D.B., Fox C.S., Black D., Ettinger B., Ernster V.L., Cummings S.R. **Hormone therapy to prevent disease and prolong life in postmenopausal women.** Ann. Intern. Med. 1992;117: 1016–1037. doi: 10.7326/0003-4819-117-12-1016.

13. Lobo R.A., Pickar J.H., Stevenson J.C., Mack W.J., Hodis H.N. **Back to the future: Hormone replacement therapy as part of a prevention strategy for women at the onset of menopause. Atherosclerosis.** 2016;254: 296–304. doi: 10.1016/j. atherosclerosis.2016.10.005.

14. **American Medical Association Guidelines for counseling post-menopausal women about preventive hormone therapy.** American College of Physicians. Ann. Intern. Med. 1992;117: 1038–1041. doi: 10.7326/0003-4819-117-12-1038.

15. Lobo R.A., Whitehead M. **Too much of a good thing? Use of progestogens in the menopause: An international consensus statement.** Fertil. Steril. 1989;51: 229–231. doi: 10.1016/ S0015-0282(16)60481-8

16. Hulley S., Grady D., Bush T., Furberg C., Herrington D., Riggs B., Vittinghoff E. **Randomized trial of estrogen plus progestin for secondary prevention of coronary heart disease in postmenopausal women**. Heart and Estrogen/progestin Replacement Study (HERS) Research Group. JAMA. 1998;280: 605–613. doi: 10.1001/jama.280.7.605.

17. Rossouw J.E., Anderson G.L., Prentice R.L., LaCroix A.Z., Kooperberg C., Stefanick M.L., Jackson R.D., Beresford S.A., Howard B.V., Johnson K.C., et al. Writing Group for the Women's Health Initiative Investigators. **Risks and benefits of estrogen plus progestin in healthy postmenopausal women: Principal results from the Women's Health Initiative randomized controlled trial.** JAMA. 2002;288: 321–333. doi: 10.1001/jama.288.3.321.

18. Anderson G.L., Limacher M., Assaf A.R., Bassford T., Beresford S.A., Black H., Bonds D., Brunner R., Brzyski R., Caan B., et al. Effects of conjugated equine estrogen in postmenopausal women with hysterectomy: The Women's Health Initiative randomized controlled trial. JAMA. 2004;291: 1701–1712. doi: 10.1001/jama.291.14.1701.

19. Hodis H.N., Wendy J.M. A window of opportunity: The reduction of coronary heart disease and total mortality with menopausal therapies is age and time dependent. Brain Res. 2011;1379: 244–252. doi: 10.1016/j.brainres.2010.10.076. [PMC free article]

20. Stuenkel C.A., Gass M.L., Manson J.E., Lobo R.A., Pal L., Rebar R.W., Hall J.E. A decade after the Women's Health Initiative—The experts do agree. Menopause. 2012;19: 846–847. doi: 10.1097/gme.0b013e31826226f2. [

21. Stevenson J.C., Hodis H.N., Pickar J.H., Lobo R.A. **Coronary heart disease, and menopause management: The swinging pendulum of HRT.** Atherosclerosis. 2009;207: 336–340. doi: 10.1016/j.atherosclerosis.2009.05.033. [

22. Manson J.E., Chlebowski R.T., Stefanick M.L., Aragaki A.K., Rossouw J.E., Prentice R.L., Anderson G., Howard B.V., Thomson C.A., LaCroix A.Z., et al. **Menopausal hormone therapy and health outcomes during the intervention and extended poststopping phases of the Women's Health Initiative randomized trials.**

JAMA. 2013;310: 1353–1368. doi: 10.1001/jama.2013.278040. [PMC free article]

23. Hsia J., Langer R.D., Manson J.E., Kuller L., Johnson K.C., Hendrix S.L., Pettinger M., Heckbert S.R., Greep N., Crawford S., et al. **Women's Health Initiative Investigators. Conjugated equine estrogens and coronary heart disease**: The Women's Health Initiative. Arch. Intern. Med. 2006;166: 357–365. doi: 10.1001/archinte.166.3.357.

24. Salpeter S.R., Walsh J.M., Greyber E., Salpeter E.E. Brief report: **Coronary heart disease events associated with hormone therapy in younger and older women. A meta-analysis.** J. Gen. Intern. Med. 2006;21: 363–366. doi: 10.1111/j.1525-1497.2006.00389. x. [PMC free article]

25. Salpeter S.R., Walsh J.M., Greyber E., Ormiston T.M., Salpeter E.E. **Mortality associated with hormone replacement therapy in younger and older women: A meta-analysis.** J. Gen. Intern. Med. 2004;19: 791–804. doi: 10.1111/j.1525-1497.2004.30281. x. [PMC free article]

26. Boardman H.M., Hartley L., Eisinga A., Main C., i Figuls M.R., Cosp X.B., Sanchez R.G., Knight B. **Hormone therapy for preventing cardiovascular disease in postmenopausal women.** Cochrane Database Syst. Rev. 2015 doi: 10.1002/14651858.CD002229.pub4.

27. Rossouw J.E., Prentice R.L., Manson J.E., Wu L., Barad D., Barnabei V.M., Ko M., LaCroix A.Z., Margolis K.L., Stefanick M.L. **Postmenopausal hormone therapy and cardiovascular disease by age and years since menopause.** JAMA. 2007;297: 1465–1477. doi: 10.1001/jama.297.13.1465.

28. Schierbeck L.L., Rejnmark L., Tofteng C.L., Stilgren L., Eiken P., Mosekilde L., Køber L., Beck Jensen J.E. **Effect of hormone replacement therapy on cardiovascular events in recently post-menopausal women:** Randomized trial. BMJ. 2012;345: e6409. doi: 10.1136/bmj. e6409.

29. Ravdin P.M., Cronin K.A., Howlader N., Berg C.D., Chlebowski R.T., Feuer E.J., Edwards B.K., Berry D.A. **The decrease in breast-cancer incidence in 2003 in the United States.** N. Engl. J. Med. 2007;356: 1670–1674. doi: 10.1056/NEJMsr070105.

30. Buist D.S., Newton K.M., Miglioretti D.L., Beverly K., Connelly M.T., Andrade S., Hartsfield C.L., Wei F., Chan K.A., Kessler L. **Hormone therapy prescribing patterns in the United States.** Obstet. Gynecol. 2004;104: 1042–1050. doi: 10.1097/01. AOG.0000143826. 38439.af.

31. Guay M.P., Dragomir A., Pilon D., Moride Y., Perreault S. **Changes in pattern use, clinical characteristics and persistence rate of hormone replacement therapy among postmenopausal women after the WHI publication.** Pharmacoepidemiol. Drug Saf. 2007;16: 17–27. doi: 10.1002/pds.1273.

32. Heitmann C., Greiser E., Dören M. **The impact of the Women's Health Initiative randomized controlled trial 2002 on perceived risk communication and use of postmenopausal hormone therapy in Germany.** Menopause. 2005;12: 405–411. doi: 10.1097/01.GME.0000153890.77135.00.

33. Clanget C., Hinke V., Lange S., Fricke R., Botko R., Pfeilschifter J. **Patterns of hormone replacement therapy in a population-based cohort of postmenopausal German women. Changes after HERS II and WHI.** Exp. Clin. Endocrinol. Diabetes. 2005;113: 529–533. doi: 10.1055/s-2005-865802.

34. Menon U., Burnell M., Sharma A., Gentry-Maharaj A., Fraser L., Ryan A., Parmar M., Hunter M., Jacobs I., UKCTOCS Group Decline in use of hormone therapy among postmenopausal women in the United Kingdom. Menopause. 2007;14: 462–467. doi: 10.1097/01.gme.0000243569.70946.9d.

35. Nelson H.D., Humphrey L.L., Nygren P., Teutsch S.M., Allan J.D. Postmenopausal Hormone Replacement Therapy: Scientific Review. JAMA. 2002;288: 872–881. doi: 10.1001/jama.288.7.872.

36. Collaborative Group on Hormonal Factors in Breast Cancer and hormone replacement therapy: Collaborative reanalyses of data from 51 epidemiological studies of 52,705 women with breast cancer and 108,411 women without breast cancer. Lancet. 1997;350: 1047–1059. doi: 10.1016/S0140-6736(97)08233-0.

37. Chlebowski R.T., Rohan T.E., Manson J.E., Aragaki A.K., Kaunitz A., Stefanick M.L., Simon M.S., Johnson K.C., Wactawski-Wende J., O'Sullivan M.J., et al. Breast cancer after use of estrogen plus

progestin and estrogen alone: Analyses of data from 2 women's health initiative randomized clinical trials. JAMA Oncol. 2015;1: 296–305. doi: 10.1001/jamaoncol.2015.0494. [PMC free article].

38. Anderson G.L., Chlebowski R.T., Rossouw J.E., Rodabough R.J., McTiernan A., Margolis K.L., Aggerwal A., David Curb J., Hendrix S.L., Allan Hubbell F., et al. **Prior hormone therapy and breast cancer risk in the Women's Health Initiative randomized trial of estrogen and progestin.** Maturitas. 2006;55: 107–115. doi: 10.1016/j.maturitas.2006.05.004.

39. Anderson G.L., Chlebowski R.T., Aragaki A.K., Kuller L.H., Manson J.E., Gass M., Bluhm E., Connelly S., Hubbell F.A., Lane D., et al. **Conjugated equine oestrogen and breast cancer incidence and mortality in postmenopausal women with hysterectomy: Extended follow-up of the Women's Health Initiative randomised placebo-controlled trial.** Lancet Oncol. 2012;13: 476–486. doi: 10.1016/S1470-2045(12)70075-X. [PMC free article].

40. Santen R.J., Yue W., Heitjan D.F. **Modeling of the growth kinetics of occult breast tumors: Role in interpretation of studies of prevention and menopausal hormone therapy.** Cancer Epidemiol. Biomark. Prev. 2012;21: 1038–1048. doi: 10.1158/1055-9965.EPI-12-0043. [PMC free article].

41. Clarke C.A., Glaser S.L., Uratsu C.S., Selby J.V., Kushi L.H., Herrinton L.J. **Recent declines in hormone therapy utilization and breast cancer incidence: Clinical and population-based evidence.** J. Clin. Oncol. 2006;24: e49–e50. doi: 10.1200/JCO.2006.08.6504.

42. Robbins A.S., Clarke C.A. **Regional changes in hormone therapy use and breast cancer incidence in California from 2001 to 2004.** J. Clin. Oncol. 2007;25: 3437–3439. doi: 10.1200/JCO.2007.11.4132.

43. Zbuk K., Anand S. **Declining incidence of breast cancer after decreased use of hormone-replacement therapy: Magnitude and time lags in different countries.** J. Epidemiol. Community Health. 2012;66: 1–7. doi: 10.1136/jech.2008.083774.

44. Katalinic A., Lemmer A., Zawinell A., Rawal R., Waldmann A. **Trends in hormone therapy and breast cancer incidence results**

from the German Network of Cancer Registries. Pathobiology. 2009;76: 90–97. doi: 10.1159/000201677.

45. Seradour B., Allemand H., Weill A., Ricordeau P. **Sustained lower rates of breast cancer incidence in France in 2007.** Breast Cancer Res. Treat. 2010;121: 799–800. doi: 10.1007/s10549-010-0779-1.

46. Canfell K., Banks E., Moa A.M., Beral V. **Decrease in breast cancer incidence following a rapid fall in use of hormone replacement therapy in Australia.** Med. J. Aust. 2008;188: 641–644.

47. De P., Neutel C.I., Olivotto I., Morrison H. **Breast cancer incidence and hormone replacement therapy in Canada.** J. Natl. Cancer Inst. 2010;102: 1489–1495. doi: 10.1093/jnci/djq345.

48. Parkin D.M. **Is the recent fall in incidence of post-menopausal breast cancer in UK related to changes in use of hormone replacement therapy?** Eur. J. Cancer. 2009;45: 1649–1653. doi: 10.1016/j.ejca.2009.01.016.

49. **A Decline in Breast-Cancer Incidence multiple letters.** N. Engl. J. Med. 2007;357: 509–513.

50. Breen N., Cronin K., Meissner H.I., Taplin S.H., Tangka F.K., Tiro J.A., McNeel T.S. **Reported drop in mammography: Is this cause for concern?** Cancer. 2007;109: 2405–2409. doi: 10.1002/cncr.22723.

51. Martin R.M., Wheeler B.W., Metcalfe C., Gunnell D. **What was the immediate impact on population health of the recent fall in hormone replacement therapy prescribing in England?** Ecological study. J. Public Health (Oxf.) 2010;32: 555–564. doi: 10.1093/pubmed/fdq021.

52. Hulley S.B., Grady D. **The WHI estrogen-alone trial–do things look any better?** JAMA. 2004;291: 1769–1771. doi: 10.1001/jama.291.14.1769.

53. Beral V., Bull D., Reeves G., **Million Women Study Collaborators Endometrial cancer and hormone-replacement therapy in the Million Women Study.** Lancet. 2005;365: 1543–1551. doi: 10.1016/S0140-6736(05)66455-0. [PubMed] [CrossRef] [Google Scholar]

54. Sjögrena L.L., Mørchb L.S., Løkkegaarda E. **Hormone replacement therapy and the risk of endometrial cancer: A systematic review.** Maturitas. 2016;91: 25–35. doi: 10.1016/j.maturitas.2016.05.013.

55. Mørch L.S., Kjaer S.K., Keiding N., Løkkegaard E., Lidegaard Ø. **The influence of hormone therapies on type I and II endometrial cancer: A nationwide cohort study**. Int. J. Cancer. 2016;138: 1506–1515. doi: 10.1002/ijc.29878.

56. Jaakkola S., Lyytinen H.K., Dyba T., Ylikorkala O., Pukkala E. **Endometrial cancer associated with various forms of postmenopausal hormone therapy: A case control study**. Int. J. Cancer. 2011;128: 1644–1651. doi: 10.1002/ijc.25762.

57. Stute P., Neulen J., Wildt L. **The impact of micronized progesterone on the endometrium: A systematic review**. Climacteric. 2016;19: 316–328. doi: 10.1080/13697137.2016.1187123.

58. Fournier A., Berrino F., Clavel-Chapelon F. **Unequal risks for breast cancer associated with different hormone replacement therapies: Results from the E3N cohort study**. Breast Cancer Res. Treat. 2008;107: 103–111. doi: 10.1007/s10549-007-9523-x. [PMC free article]

59. Fournier A., Dossus L., Mesrine S., Vilier A., Boutron-Ruault M.C., Clavel-Chapelon F., Chabbert-Buffet N. **Risks of endometrial cancer associated with different hormone replacement therapies in the E3N cohort**, 1992–2008. Am. J. Epidemiol. 2014;180: 508–517. doi: 10.1093/aje/kwu146.

60. Wachtel M.S., Yang S., Dissanaike S., Margenthaler J.A. **Hormone Replacement Therapy, likely neither Angel nor Demon**. PLoS ONE. 2015;10: e0138556. doi: 10.1371/journal.pone.0138556. [PMC free article]

61. Thurston R.C., Kuller L.H., Edmundowicz D., Matthews K.A. History of hot flashes and aortic calcification among Postmenopausal women. Menopause. 2010;17: 256–261. doi: 10.1097/gme.0b013e3181c1ad3d. [PMC free article]

62. Thurston R.C., Sutton-Tyrrell K., Everson-Rose S.A., Hess R., Powell L.H., Matthews K.A. **Hot flashes and carotid intima media thickness among midlife women**. *Menopause*. 2011;18: **352–358**. **doi: 10.1097/gme.0b013e3181fa27fd. [PMC free article]**

63. Bechlioulis A., Kalantaridou S.N., Naka K.K., Chatzikyriakidou A., Calis K.A., Makrigiannakis A., Papanikolaou O., Kaponis A., Katsouras C., Georgiou I., et al. **Endothelial function, but not**

carotid intima-media thickness, is affected early in menopause and is associated with severity of hot flushes. J. Clin. Endocrinol. Metab. 2010;95: 1199–1206. doi: 10.1210/jc.2009-2262.

64. Writing Group for the PEPI Trial Effects of estrogen or estrogen/progestin regimens on heart disease risk factors in postmenopausal women. **The Postmenopausal Estrogen/Progestin Interventions (PEPI) Trial.** JAMA. 1995;273: 199–208. doi: 10.1001/jama.1995.03520270033028.

65. Herrington D.M., Werbel B.L., Riley W.A., Pusser B.E., Morgan T.M. **Individual and combined effects of estrogen/progestin therapy and lovastatin on lipids and flow-mediated vasodilation in postmenopausal women with coronary artery disease.** J. Am. Coll. Cardiol. 1999;33: 2030–2037. doi: 10.1016/S0735-1097(99)00128-X.

66. Futterman L.G., Lemberg L. **Lp(a) lipoprotein—An independent risk factor for coronary heart disease after menopause.** Am. J. Crit. Care. 2001;10: 63–67.

67. Störk S., von Schacky C., Angerer P. **The effect of 17-estradiol on endothelial and inflammatory markers in postmenopausal women: A randomized, controlled trial.** Atherosclerosis. 2002;165: 301–307. doi: 10.1016/S0021-9150(02)00242-3.

68. Guzic-Salobir B., Keber I., Seljeflot I., Arnesen H., Vrabic L. **Combined hormone replacement therapy improves endothelial function in healthy postmenopausal women.** J. Intern. Med. 2001;250: 508–515. doi: 10.1046/j.1365-2796.2001.00910. x.

69. Wakatsuki A., Okatani Y., Ikenoue N., Fukaya T. **Effect of medroxyprogesterone acetate on endothelium-dependent vasodilation in postmenopausal women receiving estrogen.** Circulation. 2001;104: 1773–1778. doi: 10.1161/hc4001.097035.

70. Hodis H.N., Mack W.J., Henderson V.W., Shoupe D., Budoff M.J., Hwang-Levine J., Li Y., Feng M., Dustin L., Kono N., et al. **Vascular effects of early versus late postmenopausal treatment with estradiol.** N. Engl. J. Med. 2016;374: 1221–1231. doi: 10.1056/NEJMoa1505241. [PMC free article]

71. Harman S.M., Black D.M., Naftolin F., Brinton E.A., Budoff M.J., Cedars M.I., Hopkins P.N., Lobo R.A., Manson J.E., Merriam G.R.,

et al. **Arterial imaging outcomes and cardiovascular risk factors in recently menopausal women: A randomized trial.** Ann. Intern. Med. 2014;161: 249–260. doi: 10.7326/M14-0353.

72. Mikkola T.S., Tuomikoski P., Lyytinen H. **Increased cardiovascular mortality risk in women discontinuing postmenopausal hormone therapy.** J. Clin. Endocrinol. Metab. 2015;100: 4588–4594. doi: 10.1210/jc.2015-1864.

73. Kindig D.A., Cheng E.R. **Even as mortality fell in most US counties, female mortality nonetheless rose in 42.8 percent of counties from 1992 to 2006.** Health Aff. (Millwood) 2013;32: 451–458. doi: 10.1377/hlthaff.2011.0892.

74. Shetty K.D., Vogt W.B., Bhattacharya J. **Hormone replacement therapy and cardiovascular health in the United States.** Med. Care. 2009;47: 600–606. doi: 10.1097/MLR.0b013e31818bfe9b.

75. Ilesanmi-Oyelere B.L., Schollum L., Kuhn-Sherlock B., McConnell M., Mros S., Coad J., Roy N.C., Kruger M.C. **Inflammatory markers and bone health in postmenopausal women: A cross-sectional overview.** Immun. Ageing. 2019; 16:15. doi: 10.1186/s12979-019-0155-x. [PMC free article]

76. Ginaldi L., De Martinis M., Saitta S., Sirufo M.M., Mannucci C., Casciaro M., Ciccarelli F., Gangemi S. **Interleukin-33 serum levels in postmenopausal women with osteoporosis.** Sci. Rep. 2019;9: 3786. doi: 10.1038/s41598-019-40212-6. [PMC free article].

77. Banks E., Beral V., Reeves G., Balkwill A., Barnes I. **Fracture incidence in relation to the pattern of use of hormone therapy in postmenopausal women.** JAMA. 2004;291: 2212–2220. doi: 10.1001/jama.291.18.2212.

78. Grodstein F., Stampfer M.J., Falkeborn M., Naessen T., Persson I. **Post-menopausal hormone therapy and risk of cardiovascular disease and hip fracture in a cohort of Swedish women.** Epidemiology. 1999;10: 476–480. doi: 10.1097/00001648-199909000-00003.

79. Mosekilde L., Beck-Nielsen H., Sørensen O.H., Nielsen S.P., Charles P., Vestergaard P., Hermann A.P., Gram J., Hansen T.B., Abrahamsen B., et al. **Hormonal replacement therapy reduces forearm fracture incidence in recent postmenopausal women. Results of**

the Danish Osteoporosis Prevention Study. Maturitas. 2000;36: 181–193. doi: 10.1016/S0378-5122(00)00158-4.

80. Watts N.B., Cauley J.A., Jackson R.D., LaCroix A.Z., Lewis C.E., Manson J.E., Neuner J.M., Phillips L.S., Stefanick M.L., Wactawski-Wende J., et al. **Women's Health Initiative Investigators. No Increase in Fractures After Stopping Hormone Therapy: Results From the Women's Health Initiative.** J. Clin. Endocrinol. Metab. 2017;102: 302–308. doi: 10.1210/jc.2016-3270. [PMC free article].

81. Saarelainen J., Hassi S., Honkanen R., Koivumaa-Honkanen H., Sirola J., Kröger H., Komulainen M.H., Tuppurainen M. **Bone loss and wrist fractures after withdrawal of hormone therapy: The 15-year follow-up of the OSTPRE cohort.** Maturitas. 2016;85: 49–55. doi: 10.1016/j.maturitas.2015.12.011.

82. Islam S., Liu Q., Chines A., Helzner E. **Trend in the incidence of osteoporosis-related fractures among 40–to 69-year-old women: Analysis of a large insurance claims database, 2000–2005.** Menopause. 2009;16: 77–83. doi: 10.1097/gme.0b013e31817b816e.

83. Gambacciani M., Ciaponi M., Genazzani A.R. **The HRT misuse and osteoporosis epidemic: A possible future scenario.** Climacteric. 2007;10: 273–275. doi: 10.1080/13697130701511277.

84. Karim R., Dell R.M., Greene D.F., Mack W.J., Gallagher J.C., Hodis H.N. **Hip fracture in postmenopausal women after cessation of hormone therapy: Results from a prospective study in a large health management organization.** Menopause. 2011;18: 1172–1177. doi: 10.1097/gme.0b013e31821b01c7. [PMC free article].

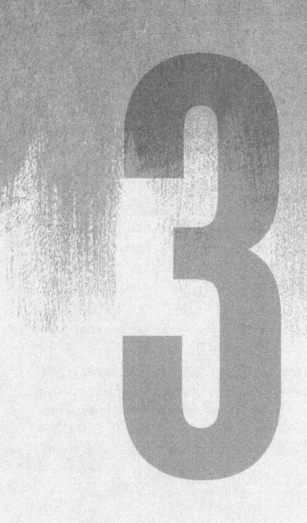

Understanding Your Hormones—The Energy Sources for Your Body

Bioidentical hormone replacement therapy (BHRT) offers new ideas about our precious gift of *life* and a state-of-the-art approach to how we can all live this experience more fully. We've shown that it's best to ignore the cacophony and noise of this rudderless ship we occupy as it drifts through evidence-based medicine. Listen to the facts. Absorb the knowledge. Exercise your *medical freedom*. Make your own call. And maybe, look for the magic place along the way.

Life is, of course, the primary topic of our narrative. All we have done, and all we will do, is about the way each of us intends to lead our lives. Go and look for the magic place, unashamed of not knowing the answers because this is new, and you are not expected to know the answers.

That speaks to our quest. It speaks to the drive of our ancestors to find the grail. It speaks to our scientists, who can always maintain sight of the power of their inquiry.

In this chapter, we'll look at the magical place.

I will offer you some enlightening information about your hormones. We'll look at insulin and its journey to a bioidentical formulation instead of using farm animals. In a special sidebar later in our narrative, I will share a complete list of the hormones that impact both the male and female bodies, and the size of that list will impress you. *(There will not be a pop quiz later.)* We have nearly fifty hormones working to make us healthy every day. I'll offer some convincing research on pellet-based bioidentical hormone replacement that involves the study of over a million patients. Then we'll review some enlightening information about testosterone studies in women.

Hormones are chemicals that coordinate different bodily functions by carrying messages through your blood to your organs, skin, muscles, and other tissues. These signals tell your body what to do and when to do it. Hormones are essential for life and your health.

Do we lose hormones as we age, or do we age because we lose hormones?

I see a bit of truth in each statement. It's hard to be definitive because we frankly do not know how many environmental toxins each of us has been exposed to, but we know that toxins damage our hormones. Regarding the loss due to age, I believe if we lived in a toxin-less environment, with clean air and water and plenty of healthy foods, no toxins, we exercised well, then our hormone levels would not change much at all as we age, even up into our nineties.

> **How many folks understand that brain fog, depressive mood, weight gain, poor sleep, loss of energy, loss of libido, and lessened zest for life represent clues of a severe loss of hormone deficiency, not a function of getting old?**

So here's the big question: If we have symptoms of hormone loss, why does our medical system not treat it without the patient begging for hormone restoration? How many folks understand that brain fog, depressive mood, weight gain, poor sleep, loss of energy, loss of libido, and lessened zest for life represent clues of a severe loss of hormone deficiency, not a function of getting old? I suspect the answer lies with the insurance industry, not the physicians.

Take your thyroid, for example. If we lose thyroid hormone as we age, most doctors treat that right away. We may disagree on what that treatment may entail (iodine, selenium, Armour Thyroid, Synthroid, etc.) But no one argues that we must treat it. The same goes for type 1 diabetes. We must treat the loss of insulin, which is a hormone. We may disagree on the treatment, but no doubt about it, we must treat. If we lose insulin, or if insulin is not made or efficient in our body, we don't say, "Diabetes is part of aging." We act. We try to lower your blood sugar somehow, either with altering chemicals and diet or giving you insulin. And now that we are not using farm animals to produce insulin, we can take advantage of the bioidentical formulation.

But when you lose gonads, which make our hormones, ovaries, or testicles, your family discussions may revolve around the idea that, "Oh. They're getting older now. It's part of aging because our culture equates gonads with sex and fertility, *which you don't need anymore after a certain age.*" Wrong.

That's why a vast majority of people think hormones mean sex hormones, these are for fertility. People forget that the key hormones estrogen, progesterone, and testosterone have four or five hundred functions. We hear, "It's common at your age." Well, it's not common.

Why not accept average? We will see the average of a sick population. Heart disease, cancer, Alzheimer's, dementia, osteoporosis, and diabetes, are epidemic. *Her symptoms are common for her age.* No. Failure to treat hormone loss will not have a good ending. I do not want what is common to my population. And I will not accept that

65

notion for my patients. I want optimal. And not just optimal for my age. I want optimal, as in the best I ever have been.

I do not want what is common to my population. And I will not accept that notion for my patients. I want optimal. And not just optimal for my age. I want optimal, as in the best I ever have been.

Every cell has a life expectancy before it goes into senescence (the process of deterioration by age) and dies off by apoptosis, but we're speeding that process up faster and faster and faster by not responding to the clues.

The Cleveland Clinic defines hormones like this: "Hormones are chemical messengers that coordinate different functions in your body. Several glands, organs, and tissues make and release hormones, many of which make up your endocrine system. Scientists have identified over fifty hormones in the human body so far."[68]

Most of the tissues (mainly glands) that create and release them make up your endocrine system. Hormones control many different bodily processes, including:

- Metabolism
- Homeostasis (constant internal balance), such as blood pressure and blood sugar regulation, fluid (water) and electrolyte balance, and body temperature
- Growth and development
- Sexual function
- Reproduction
- Sleep-wake cycle
- Mood

With hormones, a little bit goes a long way. Because of this, minor changes in levels can cause significant changes to your body and lead to certain conditions that require medical treatment.

Often, a bodily process involves a chain reaction of several different hormones.[69] A hormone will only act on a part of your body if it "fits"—if the cells in the target tissue have receptors that receive the message of the hormone. Think of a hormone as a key and the cells of its target tissue, such as an organ or fat tissue, as specially shaped locks. If the hormone fits the lock (receptor) on the cell wall, then it'll work; the hormone will deliver a message that causes the target site to take a specific action.

Your body uses hormones for two types of communication. The first type involves communication between two endocrine glands: one gland releases a hormone, which stimulates another gland to change the levels of hormones that it's releasing. An example of this is the communication between your pituitary gland and thyroid. Your pituitary gland releases thyroid-stimulating hormone (TSH), which triggers your thyroid gland to release its hormones, affecting various aspects of your body.[70]

The second type of communication occurs between an endocrine gland and a target organ. An example is when your pancreas releases insulin, which then acts on your muscles and liver to help process glucose.

THE CAT'S OUT OF THE BAG

The *cat's out of the bag* about my preference for pellet therapy. It works beautifully. It's all we do. I believe we are the only hormone replacement practice in the nation that only uses bioidentical pellets. It's interesting where that idiom about the cat originated. We use it in a fun way to describe a secret being revealed (whimsically).

The origin of this saying is disputed, but the most common explanation I could find suggests that it came from a trick used in the past in English marketplaces. Apparently, at an earlier time in history, baby pigs were often sold at the market. The seller would give the buyer the piglet in a bag. As a trick to save money, the seller would sometimes stick a cat in the bag rather than a piglet. The buyer might not realize he had been cheated until the cat came out of the bag and the trick was revealed.[71]

I must say that this story reminds me of synthetic hormones.

Synthetic hormones can quite likely be animal-based, leading to differences in molecular structure from endogenous hormones. The cat's out of the bag there too. The trick has been revealed. Synthetic hormones are chemically altered and not identical to human hormones. For example, the popular estrogen-replacement drug Premarin is made from horse urine. Release the horses.

THE STORY OF THE HORSES

One of the most important distinctions I can make when explaining the breakthrough research that has been done for bioidentical hormones is to tell the story of the horses.

I used synthetic hormones for years in my OB/GYN practice, especially as a remedy for menopause. But I greeted the development of bioidentical hormones made from plants with open arms.

Back in the 1930s, Canadian scientists discovered that the urine of pregnant mares was beneficial for manufacturing water-soluble estrogens, or synthetic hormones. Now we needed this at the time. Entrepreneurial ranchers began to pop up, especially in Canada, nicknaming it "equine ranching," collecting "PMU" (pregnant mares' urine). The drugs were approved both in the United States and Canada in the 1940s.[72]

As the pharmaceutical industry began to fine-tune the production of synthetic hormones, there was a burst of interest in the 1980s and 1990s. This spiked demand and resulted in over five hundred ranches, mainly in Canada, where they harvested the urine from thousands of pregnant horses. Today, the market has greatly lessened due to the rocky road of clinical research, but larger and better-developed PMU ranches number about nineteen under contract with Pfizer.[73]

This is how one of the most widely prescribed drugs in America is made from animal waste. The drug is Premarin, cleverly named after "'pregnant mares' urine," an estrogen-therapy drug currently manufactured by Pfizer (formerly Wyeth Pharmaceuticals), which also produces Prempro, an estrogen/progestin combination. Both drugs contain pregnant mares' urine (PMU).

For most of their eleven-month pregnancies, ranchers confine these horses to small stalls so that they cannot turn around or take more than a single step in any direction. Current guidelines state, "no smaller than 4'x12,'" and the animals must wear rubber urine-collection bags (called "boots") at all times, which, according to watchdog groups, causes chafing and lesions. Ranchers regulate their drinking water so that their urine will yield more concentrated estrogen. After the birth of the foals, the horses are impregnated again, and this cycle continues for about twelve years. Official guidelines suggest allowing the mares to walk around twice a week in a corral.[74]

With so much revenue from this new hormone therapy, drug companies promoted these synthetic drugs extensively to women and gynecologists during the last decades of the twentieth century, especially touting its protection for the heart.

Marketing efforts worked. By 1992, Premarin was the number one prescribed drug in the United States. By 1997, its sales exceeded $1 billion.[75]

Usage of these drugs plummeted after a 2002 study warned women of the side effects and risks of developing breast cancer and other complications from these synthetic hormones.[76]

Animal welfare groups continually monitor this industry.

The People for the Ethical Treatment of Animals (PETA) website takes a dim view of this PMU practice. They cite commentary from Katherine Swing, MD, a board-certified Obstetrician and Gynecologist and Diplomate of the American Board of Obesity Medicine.

"There is ample literature to support the safety, efficacy, and better side effect profiles of bioidentical hormones, such as estradiol, progesterone, and testosterone, over synthetic hormones, such as Premarin and Prempro," Dr. Swing noted.[77]

You know, if we developed all the benefits of hormone replacement onto a single pill, a pill that would decrease belly fat, lower diabetes, reduce metabolic syndrome, increase libido, decrease dementia, decrease Alzheimer's, strengthen bone, protect the heart, decrease prostate cancer, improve mood, help develop muscle, and decrease breast cancer, what would it be worth?

Would it be priceless?

We have that. It's just not a pill because Big Pharma cannot patent a natural molecule that restores your youthful biological chemistry. Plus, such a pill would lose much of its potency, passing through the digestive system.

We're not happy with human remedies that we create from the waste products of animals, yet this has been a way of life for science to test out drugs and therapies over the past fifty years.

If we somehow released the horses from their slavery and restraint, physicians would drop the synthetics and probably prescribe oral estradiol, which is good. That's what I used before bioidentical came along.

The problem with oral administration is that the body absorbs just 2–5 percent. (Even the most current method, which deploys the hormones through the lymphatic system of the intestinal tract, only produces 3–5 percent.) And as it passes through the liver, it can cause complications such as increased blood pressure and blood clots. What does the molecule do when it's in the liver? It increases blood clots in the coagulation factors. That's the problem with drugs taken orally. If we use injections, we have to prepare for peaks and valleys of impact, and most injections are not bioidentical. Some injectables, such as testosterone undecanoate, can have a serious risk of side effects.

HORMONE TREATMENT OPTIONS

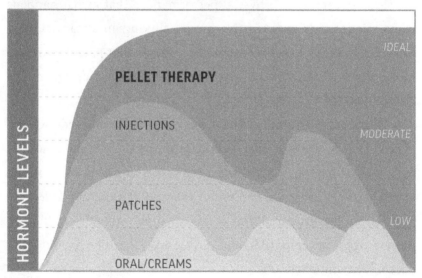

Creams could be used, but the skin is not an excellent absorbent over time. When we put pellets in subcutaneous fat, it mimics the ovary; it mimics the testicle. So, the best way to mimic the human body physiologically, anatomically, and endocrinologically would be to put time-release pellets in fat.

THE DANGERS OF SYNTHETIC ANABOLIC STEROIDS

While the astounding science marches forward, revealing wonderful impacts of BHRT on disorders of the brain, it is important to understand that the widespread abuse of anabolic steroids in the sporting world involved synthetic hormones, not bioidentical.

All this came about when the pharmaceutical industry began to make chemical modifications to the testosterone molecule, seeking to improve its pharmacological effects. *Voilà!* Anabolic steroids were born, which found their way under the table to be abused by recreational and professional athletes searching for improvements in physical appearance or physical performance. That's what happens when science tries to better Nature by altering an already-perfect molecule in order to patent medicines. You cannot patent a natural molecule. Nor can you improve on what God has designed. It's already perfect.

"Illicit use of anabolic AS has been correlated with several adverse effects, such as cardiovascular, endocrine, reproductive, and neurobehavioral dysfunctions," noted the authors of a landmark study in the recent book *Sex Hormones in Neurodegenerative Processes and Diseases*.[78]

"Given the structural similarities, Anabolic Steroids can bind to the androgenic receptor (AR) and exert testosterone-like physiological effects," the authors note.[79]

So far, science has identified three classes of AS. Three ways to ruin your body. Illicit use of AS is characterized by administration of doses ten to one thousand times higher than the doses prescribed to treat medical conditions.

The first class includes injectable AS with esterification of the 17B-hydroxl group on testosterone molecule, such as testosterone propionate.

The second class of AS is composed by injectable steroids, although using the biologically active compound is the 19-nor-testosterone, instead of testosterone.

The third class includes C17-alkylated AS, such as 17α-methyltestosterone (MET), oxymetholone, methandrostenolone, and stanozolol. Given that these drugs can be orally administered, the effects are relatively weaker compared to the C-17-alkylated compounds.[80]

These abused drugs cause lasting damage to the body and mind. Abusers are risking significant impairment. (There's more on anabolic steroid abuse in chapter 8.)

Bioidentical hormones are man-made, derived from plants, often soy and yams, chemically identical to the human body—binding to estrogen and testosterone receptors in the same way endogenous hormones have.

The FDA approved some forms of manufactured bioidentical hormones, including estrogens and progesterone, however, the FDA has not approved custom-compounded bioidentical hormones.

There is a 75-milligram testosterone pellet approved by the FDA in 2008. It has three ingredients, two of which are bioidentical, 17-beta testosterone and steric acid (as a binder). The third one is synthetic, polyvinylpyrrolidone USP 2 mg, which is registered with the EPA as a hazardous material and may be toxic to human skin.

It is that component that makes it patentable. Pharmaceutical companies cannot patent organic molecules.

BIOIDENTICAL PELLET PLACEMENT

BHRT can be administered via cream, suppository, oral medication, or injection. At Optimal Bio, pellets the size of a grain of rice are the preferred method of hormone replacement delivery, as they mimic natural hormones best and keep them dosed at a steady state. Pellets are implanted into fatty tissues of the lower lateral buttocks or lower back and side and can last for several months. Patients typically feel the impact of pellets within three weeks of the first implant—there's no substitute for pellet therapy.

Women are more susceptible to feeling the effects of a hormonal imbalance. A drop in testosterone and estrogen could be subtle over the years; however, once menopause occurs, a woman's estrogen levels drop significantly, some to zero, causing extreme symptoms.

The male body is more resilient; however, low testosterone can cause many physical issues over time. Men have a steady drop in their testosterone levels from their twenties onward and a drastic reduction in their forties and fifties, which is now referred to as "andropause" (the male equivalent to menopause).

Women typically require pellets every three to five months, while men need them every four to six months.

Getting started with BHRT involves an in-person consultation with your hormone replacement medical providers to discuss your health concerns and treatment options. This will be followed up with lab (blood) work. You can have your lab work done anywhere close to your home. Our practice uses an algorithm based on your specific lab results, health history, and symptoms, including your gender, physique, and overall activity, to develop your hormone therapy plan. Once an individualized plan has been finalized, your first pellet procedure will be scheduled. The painless process takes only a few moments. You will wear a compression of ice over the tiny incision for a few days to minimize discomfort when the lidocaine wears off.

One of the breakthroughs in bioidentical science revolutionized insulin. Insulin from cattle and pigs was used for many years to treat diabetes and saved millions of lives, but it caused allergic reactions in many patients. The first genetically engineered, synthetic "human" insulin was produced in 1978 using E. coli bacteria to produce the insulin. *Brilliant.* They had bacteria that took our DNA and recombinant DNA and made insulin. Biosynthetic human insulin (BHI) produced by recombinant DNA technology has been proven identical to human pancreatic insulin. It differs from pork insulin in one carboxy-terminal amino acid of the B-chain, where alanine substitutes for threonine. Release the pigs and cattle now.

But now that bioidentical hormones are available and much better in every way, pharmaceutical revenue and nineteen Canadian ranchers are the only hang-ups from switching to bioidentical, plant-based hormones.

In a brilliant essay entitled "The Wild History of Women's Hormone Therapy," writer Meryl Davids Landau of *Everyday Health* describes the historical context.

"Hormone therapy has had its ups and downs, creating confusion for women seeking relief from hot flashes or vaginal dryness. Which is a shame," says Stephanie Faubion, MD, the director of the Center for Women's Health at Mayo Clinic and the medical director of the North American Menopause Society (NAMS), "because the science is clear that for most women, the benefits of menopausal hormone therapy (HT) for symptom relief outweigh any risks."[81]

How did we get all the misperceptions about hormone therapy that still muddle decision-making about HT? We have landmark studies that scared everybody and were thoroughly discredited years later. We have a governmental medical system asleep at the wheel, having issued just one pitiful regulatory review of compounded bioidentical hormone therapy. At the same time, two decades of advancements never slowed a bit.

We have pharmaceutical companies clinging to their jaw-dropping capacity for sticking to animal-based formulations. We have insurance companies dictating what clinical remedies doctors can use. Mix all this up, stir well, and then along comes bioidentical hormone therapy, made from plant cells, and almost all the side effects and adverse effects of synthetic (*think horse urine*) hormone replacement no longer show up.

Meanwhile, folks have several choices.

The first choice is to wait until our governmental leadership catches up with the breakthroughs before we take advantage of the power of bioidentical hormone replacement therapy. The risk is not doing anything while your body continues to react to the loss of hormones.

The second choice might be to let your voice be heard in your insurance company or your elected representatives. Good luck with that.

The third and better choice is to exercise your medical liberty. It's your life; perhaps you can make better decisions than insurance executives or politicians. That's the choice that we'll discuss further in the next chapter: to decide that our desire to age gracefully is more powerful than our desire to be controlled.

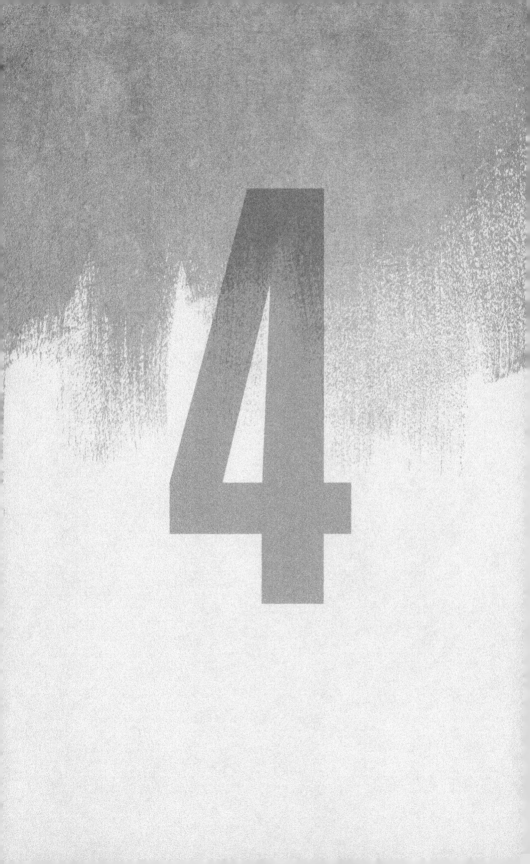

Medical Liberty
Is a Verb—
How Well-Intended Ideas
Become Stupid Rules

A nother instinct common among Americans today is the historical love of liberty. We have always been willing to fight for our liberty. When you can access a solution to the frailty of aging, and governmental authorities stop you for no good reason, you now understand what we mean by "medical liberty." This notion ties into the powerful thinking of our nation's founders.

In 1855, during the tense political years before the War between the States, Thomas Bangs Thorpe, a patriot, produced a book called *A Voice to America* to remind Americans that we have something precious.

"It is too important a truth for any of us to overlook, that the American Republic is the home of Liberty, and the final hope of the world … We hold the treasure in our keeping; we are the trustees of a possession that is to enrich mankind."[82]

As soon as we bump up against the effects of aging, we feel we cannot control them; we are told, "That's normal; it's common." Well, it's not normal, and it's no longer common. It's now preventable.

I bring this up because I have cared for over twenty thousand patients, and almost every one had to decide to choose BHRT independently of government or insurance guidance. The FDA has been asleep at the wheel, doing episodic "watchful waiting" for over two decades, and insurance companies have failed to see the flood of evidence supporting BHRT and youthful wellness in our later years. Many men do not even know their testosterone score, and many women are not even aware of the presence of this vital hormone. Neither is on a standard blood panel. You must ask for an extra test. So what do you do? We decide for ourselves, not looking for control and guidance from the well-meaning but overgrown medical-industrial complex.

> The US Food and Drug Administration (FDA) has shown only marginal interest in providing the American public with unbiased, helpful information about compounded bioidentical hormones: one study and a fact sheet in sixteen years.
>
> The FDA has approved dozens of hormone therapy products for men and women, including estrogen, progesterone, testosterone, and related compounds, but because well-controlled clinical trials are thin on the topic of bioidentical, holistic options, this giant federal agency jumped into action.
>
> In the fall of 2018, The FDA commissioned the National Academies to create a consensus study report they named "The Clinical Utility of Compounded Bioidentical Hormone Therapy: A Review of Safety, Effectiveness, and Use."
>
> Here's what this multiorganizational study concluded in their 2020 release of this 320-page publication:

"For the large patient population using cBHT (compounded bioidentical hormone therapy) it is difficult, if not impossible, for clinicians to provide evidence-based guidance on the safety and effectiveness of each unique formulation." [83]

Despite not having solid, evidence-based research on the new bioidentical hormones, most of the book (with an eye-catching full-color cover) was brainstorming how the government could outline a comprehensive surveillance and regulatory framework, gather data, regulate physicians, pharmacists, manufacturers, medical boards, professional societies, schools of pharmacy, marketing regulations, labeling, formula approvals, strengthen state oversight, reporting systems, and research.

The entire study can be vulnerable to criticism. The study methods describe a search strategy "to produce an evidence-based body of research that could inform its work." This resulted in 16,874 articles in the English language, "which was reduced to 11,224 articles with potential relevance to the committee's charge." Applying their keyword criteria to that list produced less than fifty articles to review.[84]

The last time the FDA weighed in on bioidentical was in 2008, when they released a publication, "Bioidenticals: Sorting Myths from Facts" dispelling the myths of bioidenticals, which led with the fact that this new development is not-FDA recognized. The phrase "We are not aware of ..." is frequently used in the publication.

The FDA Question:

This 2020 consensus report examines the clinical utility and uses of cBHT drug preparations and reviews the available evidence that would support marketing claims of the safety and effectiveness of cBHT preparations. It also assesses whether the available evidence suggests that these preparations have clinical utility and safety profiles warranting their clinical use and identifies patient populations that might benefit from cBHT preparations in lieu of FDA-approved BHT."

The FDA Answer:

Well-designed and properly controlled clinical trials are needed.

Our government, which could, in a single graceful motion, make this available to millions of people, has not disapproved of BHRT, but it hasn't approved it either. Two reports on it in sixteen years do not make a believer out of me. Instead of tracking a breakthrough in clinical excellence, they can't seem to get away from making financially motivated clinical judgments for the physicians. The pharmaceutical and insurance corporations follow the government and exercise way too much control over our doctors' *medical freedom*. Unfortunately, they seem to make determinations based solely on finance, not necessarily on what physicians decide to prescribe for the patient.

Testosterone is the most abundant biologically active gonadal hormone throughout the female life span. However, unfortunately, due to misconceptions, women remain without any FDA-approved testosterone therapies, while more than thirty approved testosterone therapies have been created for men. This has resulted in millions of women suffering in silence with prevalent symptoms that could quickly be addressed with testosterone.

The cat's out of the bag again.

For a decade, we have improved the process, helped redesign the bioidentically pure pellet, and innovated a new subcutaneous insertion technique.

WHY WE HAVE LOST OUR HORMONES

I want to digress for a moment and address the elephant in the room: why we have lost our hormones over time. One of the most brilliant business leaders I have ever worked with is Jim Baker. He shared a letter with me he wrote several years ago explaining why he and his wife chose to make BHRT part of their formula for quality of life.

Jim and Colleen Baker share their BHRT experience and an eye-opening analysis of why we have lost our hormones. Jim has spent the last thirty years in the business world as an entrepreneur, investor, and advisor. He wrote this letter for Dr. Robert Malone, MD, MA, a world-famous scientist, physician, writer, podcaster, commentator, and advocate. Dr. Malone is a believer in our fundamental freedom of free speech.

He played an early consultant/advisory role in the development of a traditional vaccine that employed protein subunits of spike and the nucleocapsid. Author of *Lies My Government Told Me: And the Better Future Coming* (2023), Dr. Malone's open testimony appears later in this chapter.

Dr. Malone asked Jim to recall his BHRT experience for his website. Jim also points out the many scientific reasons why our hormones diminish, and that list of toxins will sweep away your notions that it just means you're just getting old. Jim has since joined our practice and is using his business mastery to lead us into national prominence.

A SPECIAL MESSAGE TO MEN AND WOMEN ABOUT RESTORING YOUR HORMONES
Do You Want to Be Average?

Jim Baker, principal, Optimal Bio, and author of *The Adventure Begins When The Plan Falls Apart: Converting a Crisis into Company Success*

I didn't think I was average a few years ago.

As a devoted father of four, a loving husband, and an entrepreneur who had a successful exit from a clinical trials business, I have built myself upon the goal of achieving excellence in every facet of my life. I strive to be better every day, whether as a husband, father, or business owner. However, I needed good health to reach this goal of mine; my body had to serve as a tool rather than an obstacle in my journey toward excellence. Because of this, I have always tried my best to eat healthily, exercise six days a week, monitor my alcohol intake, and follow traditional medical advice.

My wife, Colleen, has always tried to live in a healthy manner as well. However, several years ago, she began experiencing significant menopausal symptoms that were quite debilitating. My wife was a former patient of a highly respected OB/GYN in Cary, North Carolina. She learned that after his sale, he had opened a new practice focusing on wellness which takes a whole-body approach of balancing the body through bioidentical hormone replacement therapy (BHRT), thyroid, adrenal, and traditional wellness therapy. Following a consultation and lab work, my wife became a perfect candidate for hormone replacement. Soon after Colleen began receiving treatment and taking preventative measures to balance her hormones, her menopausal symptoms disappeared, and she felt like her healthy self again. At the risk of sounding cliché, I believe her life had changed for the better.

All the while, however, I was still living in this illusion of being above average or excellent when it came to my health and all things physical (except when it came to my golf game). Yet I couldn't help but think that I, like my wife, could also benefit from balancing my hormones and my body, thus bettering my well-being altogether. However, despite my wife's experience, I needed to do my own research to be convinced that I had room to improve my well-being.

My research started with the goal of answering two questions: What exactly causes our hormones to become imbalanced in the first place, and just how many people are affected by hormone imbalance? To my shock, I discovered a multitude of things could be causing hormonal imbalances. I also discovered that it wasn't just my wife suffering from hormone imbalances.

After some research, I found that on average, the testosterone levels in both men and women are three to four times less than what they would have been thirty years ago. This was shocking, as it meant that most of our population, whether male or female, unknowingly struggles with a hormonal imbalance. This led me to get my own hormones tested, and I was shocked to find that at age fifty-four, my hormone levels tested at 286, whereas my father at age fifty-four would have tested close to 1,000. After receiving these test results, I began to dig further, asking *why* the decrease in hormone levels.

This means that the dangerous chemicals in PVC piping affects our entire population, regardless of age or gender.

As America has become one of the top-medicated countries in the world, the decline in hormone levels may result from certain medications we take. Scientists are still debating whether or not the use of statins reduces testosterone significantly.

Another common cause of hormone imbalance is sugar consumption. Unfortunately, while a lot of Americans may think they have a healthy diet, many individuals just consume "unhealthy health foods," high in sugar.

Researchers from Massachusetts General Hospital in Boston have found that glucose ingestion was associated with a significant decrease in the male hormone testosterone. The study, published in the journal *Clinical Endocrinology*, shows that 75 grams of sugar intake causes a 25 percent drop in testosterone levels for up to two hours after consumption.[85]

A lack of sleep can cause hormone imbalance as well. Our bodies were designed to get consistent, quality sleep. When you don't sleep well, it throws off your body, resulting in a decrease in testosterone. Sleep is important for plenty of reasons. What you might not have known is that sleep impacts your hormones, and hormone levels impact sleep.

Sleep affects many hormones in the body, including those related to stress or hunger.

Too much and not enough time under the covers can influence hormones. That's why a good night's sleep is essential to keeping your hormones balanced.[86]

Environmental toxins represent another cause of hormonal imbalance, such as air fresheners, perfumes, and pesticides. The world is waking up to the danger of exposure to many people living around the agricultural areas, farms and manufacturing and processing plants of glyphosate. In agricultural areas and farms, farmers and gardeners can be exposed to glyphosate via inhalation, dermal contact and/or ocular contact while using glyphosate.[87]

Heavy metals such as aluminum and mercury are hazardous to humans and can also cause hormone imbalance when they build up in the body. Do you know the most common way those chemicals get into our bodies? We surmise that amalgam mercury dental fillings might rank up there, or the general environment, but most folks would not guess also through standard vaccines. This makes you wonder: Is this why, despite being the most vaccinated country in the world, there are still thirty-three other nations with lower infant mortality rates than the United States?

Thimerosal, a mercury-based preservative, has been used for decades in the United States in multidose vials (vials containing more than one dose) of medicines and vaccines. There is no evidence of harm caused by the low doses of thimerosal in vaccines, except for minor reactions like redness and swelling at the injection site. However, in July 1999, the Public Health Service agencies, the American Academy of Pediatrics, and vaccine manufacturers agreed that thimerosal should be reduced or eliminated in vaccines as a precautionary measure.[88]

And mercury as a toxin is being globally studied by over 140 nations in the Minamata Convention.[89]

Conducting my research, coupled with a quest to be above average, brought me to the decision to receive BHRT. I have not regretted the decision.

What sets BHRT apart from synthetic hormone treatments and the creams, shots, and oral treatments is its efficacy and adverse event (it works with zero or minimal side effects) profile. The all-natural bioequivalent hormone pellet that's been around since the mid-1930s and has been proven safe and effective. It differs from the synthetic pellet as it is plant-based (yam, soy, olive oil) and bioequivalent to your body.

As our hormone provider states, "Testosterone is your body's engine oil where the engine oil and filter in your car were designed to lubricate and protect other parts from contaminants and wear. But over time, those elements become thin and no longer protect the same way. Have you noticed how your car engine sounds different when you start it after you have run it four thousand miles on the same oil? Only after you change the oil will your car return to optimal performance. Changing your car's oil every five thousand to seventy-five hundred miles (except in rare cases) is crucial to its health."

Our bodies function the same way. Over time, hormone levels decrease, and they must be renewed and restored. The pellet replacement therapy starts with an initial insertion where the pellets are placed underneath the epidermis in the fat part of your backside. It is a straightforward ten-minute procedure done in the office. Each pellet placement lasts four to six months until your body needs another oil change. After beginning my therapy, I have noticed how well I feel through day-to-day life, workouts, and in everything I do.

I believe in *medical freedom*, and that discipline equals freedom. Unfortunately, when seeking traditional medical solutions, we don't always have a choice: we receive a drug to treat a symptom, and our aches and pains are chalked up to be a result of lifestyle or age. While traditional medical solutions may mitigate our symptoms, they generally place limits on our bodies and fail to treat our actual ailment. You must see a whole-body approach to healthcare, where providers listen and then treat the cause, not the symptom. BHRT has completely transformed my health for the better, which in turn gives me the ability to stay disciplined in every aspect of my life, thus allowing me to better myself every day.

If you are like me and Colleen, you want to have choices as you get older, which will provide the freedom to live life to the fullest.

If we want to travel, we want the freedom to walk or ride a bike and not sit in a tour bus all day.

If we want to see mountains, we want the freedom to hike to the top to see the view. If we want to exercise with our adult kids, we like the freedom to run instead of walk with them. I hope that most of you would like the same. It's your body, and you only get one. Seek knowledge and learn why all of us are becoming sicker and sicker. Most importantly, be your own person and do what's best for you.

Do you still want to be average?

—Jim Baker

For a decade, we have improved the process, helped redesign the bioidentically pure pellet, and innovated a new subcutaneous insertion technique where our patients hardly feel a thing. We have created a unique tool that inserts the pellets in only a few seconds, and liberal use of lidocaine eliminates the discomfort. These new innovative techniques deliver natural bioidentical hormones within the purest, most natural pellets, gently inserted under the skin of the hip, releasing desperately needed hormones into the body for months. I have been mastering the blood chemistry and our algorithm (the formula of the pellets), which we customize for every patient based on their blood work, sex, age, and health history.

I go by the procedures developed by a pioneer in the field, Abraham Morgentaler, MD, FACS, author of the 2008 groundbreaking book *Testosterone for Life*. To make the pellet insertion experience almost painless, I innovated a few things: I add sodium bicarbonate and epinephrine to the lidocaine numbing agent, which takes away the burning sensation when we do the pellet insertion. I also chose a better location for the pellets. Going more lateral or upward is where you're trained, which is a good space, but I was just thinking about the anatomy. I knew if I went down toward the femur head, there's more space there, and all of us have a little bit of fat there to secure the placement. Finally, we tape ice on immediately and make the compression bandage tight, a technique we have mastered now that takes the discomfort away.

Millions of men and women across America have experienced BHRT, and they love it. *Medical freedom* rears its head, and the powerful word-of-mouth testimony overrides our oracles' double-talk in insurance and government. These BHRT recipients, which includes thousands of our patients, are doing precisely what they should do. Without trustworthy guidance from our regulators, they say, *we'll make the call, thank you very much.* And by the way, that's how it should be. Our desire for youthful aging is stronger than our desire to be controlled.

> **Our desire for youthful aging is stronger than our desire to be controlled.**

Ten years after that cold winter morning in 2012, our BHRT practice cared for our twenty thousandth patient. My staff read out the results like a winning box score.

We recheck blood chemistry and hormone levels after thirty days and adjust the supplements we have suggested as necessary. We consider another pellet insertion three to five months later based on the results. This is pure science. It's not luck. No guesswork. No quest to prepare for. No fountain to sip from. This defines liberty, folks—medical *liberty*. And every American deserves it.

The effects of this new restorative therapy must be shared. This new choice should be available to everyone. I believe that our future wellness hangs in the balance. Your freedom goes away when you don't have it. Unlike many of the advanced breakthroughs emerging in America and around the developing world, I insisted that we provide this therapy at a price point that ordinary people will be willing to afford. Part of my medical freedom, an important part, rests in my ability to set fees within reach of most working Americans. Many miracle drugs and medicines are so expensive that only the wealthiest can afford them. Insurers play a waiting game. *Sure, there's something better out there, but not for you.*

PATIENT OUTCOMES

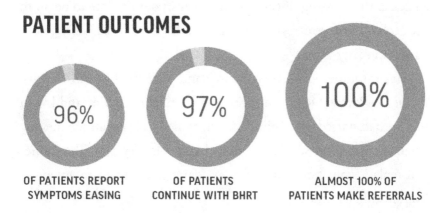

96%	97%	100%
OF PATIENTS REPORT SYMPTOMS EASING	OF PATIENTS CONTINUE WITH BHRT	ALMOST 100% OF PATIENTS MAKE REFERRALS

Ongoing ten-year patient outcomes report, Optimal Bio, published January 2023

BHRT is not new, but most people have not heard about it yet. Everyone has heard about testosterone, estrogen, and progesterone. Most folks associate this with skin creams, salves, and needles. I would compare the two as the difference between adding a quart of oil to your car versus getting an entire oil change, filter, and spark plugs, and, yes, cleaning the windows.

Most patients come to us tired of being tired. Many are experiencing anxiety, depression, mood swings, muscle pain, poor libido, brain fog, and a serious lack of energy. We all have an array of hormones. They provide the power for our body's energy. Simply stated, as we age, our hormones drain away. The loss of hormones in men and women represents the beginning of the dying process.

Because bioidentical hormone pellets are plant-based, using cells that are precisely like natural body cells that dissolve. The rate of testosterone release has been measured at 1.3 mg/day for the 200-mg pellet and 0.65 mg/day for the 100-mg pellet.[90] They provide hormone restoration over time, just as your body naturally would replace the needed hormones.

I decided to write *Restore* to broaden this message and offer you a peek at the most significant opportunity in our lifetime to begin to age gracefully. If we can get the culture's attention, we can change our nation in many ways.

It's the time between right now and your final breath that we discuss in *Restore.* Do not miss the opportunity. Both Jody and I wish that we had started this regimen much earlier. Jody began the therapy when she was forty-seven. I began when I was fifty-one. The sooner you replace your hormones, the less damage is done to your body from insufficient fuel.

You can miss this moment for any reason you wish. But please do not let the reason be that your government hasn't told you it's OK. They are not good at managing new things. Do not wait until your insurance company has figured out how to dictate where, when, and how much of any medical remedy you can receive. Do not wait for Big Pharma to rule on which tier the bioidentical pellets fall into.

In addition to not relying on our government to guide your decision-making, please do not let friends and family discourage your decision. It is your decision. Your *medical freedom.* People who know nothing about it will probably chirp. The line between naivete and cynicism is very thin. Do your homework. Make the call.

Medical doctors give you the information you need to make your own medical choices., to exercise your medical liberty. I quit taking insurance because they were paying me too much money and demanding that I practice restorative medicine under their direction—which began as soon as I accepted a contract from them. I wouldn't say I like their value proposition. I start to bristle the moment they walk in the door.

The government should have absolutely nothing to do with the practice of medicine, and one day, we all have to ask them to stand down. Most of us are anesthetized to it, until this overreach starts to affect our life, our health, and the quality of our care.

We are supposed to fuss a bit if we follow the warnings and advice of our country's earliest leaders and European observers of this Republic. (They used much stronger and more interesting language than "fuss.") Three-quarters of a century after our founding, a brilliant Frenchman published his observations and championed liberty.

> *Away, then, with quacks and organizers. Away with their rings, and their chains, and their hooks, and their pinchers! Away with their artificial methods! Away with their social laboratories, their governmental whims, their centralization, their tariffs ... And now, after having vainly inflicted upon the social body so many systems, let them end where they ought to have begun—reject all systems and try liberty— liberty, which is an act of faith in God and His work.[91]*

—FRÉDÉRIC BASTIAT, 1850

In my practice, we are setting an example of personalized medicine— a simple premise. You are in control. We are here to advise. We will inform you of our hopes for you, give you our best advice, and then you do whatever you choose. There's nobody, no company, no bureaucratic snarl, no faceless authority, between you and me. We will never second-guess your choice. People are looking for this kind of liberty and freedom. My patients are grateful for this. They sense that this is how it should be. Once they experience this kind of medicine, they do not want to go back to everything being controlled by middlemen.

Here's brief testimony from a scientist who had a big hand in inventing the mRNA and DNA vaccines. On March 24, 2022,

Robert Malone, MD, MS, wrote of his experience with bioidentical hormone replacement on his website in "Who Is Robert Malone?"[92] Dr. Malone is the author of *Lies My Government Told Me: And the Better Future Coming* (2023):

> A few years ago, before all of this "global crisis" began, I had really started to slow down and was settling into a glide path toward retirement. Travel, as well as many other things in life, had lost its luster. My wife Jill was worried about the effects of aging on both of us and the loss of bone density that had plagued her mother. As she usually does, she took on this challenge with a vengeance and was not going to give up without a fight.
>
> Digging into the literature, she discovered that the whole story regarding hormone replacement therapy was a lot more complicated than we had been led to believe.
>
> Many, both younger and older, were discovering a sort of second life with careful medical management of key hormones, and data were demonstrating that this can have a huge impact on postmenopausal bone density deterioration in women. So, off we went into the world of bioidentical hormone replacement.
>
> As we have been traveling all over the country, particularly in the various Florida medical communities which serve a more elderly population, we have encountered many physicians and medical care providers that have extolled the benefits of careful management of hormone levels. I have been personally amazed at the vitality of those who are receiving this type of treatment and have also been amazed

at the difference it has made in our own lives. We just feel younger, have more stamina, and are able to maintain a schedule that we could not have sustained a decade ago.

Please keep in mind that the biggest risks for developing severe Covid include obesity and diabetes. This is the underlying epidemic that has driven much of the death and disease associated with SARS-CoV-2. And one of the best things that you can do to prevent severe disease is to live a healthy life, lose weight, keep your blood sugar under control, and make sure that your vitamin D levels are well above 50 nanograms per milliliter.

A couple of weeks ago, we went in for our checkup and oil change at the Charlottesville clinic, which we have come to rely on, and ran into a highly respected clinical research colleague who has also had his life transformed by this treatment. We talked for a while, compared stories. And I asked if he would be interested in writing a guest piece for our substack.[93]

(Note: Jim Baker's message "Do You Want to Be Average" appeared earlier in this chapter.)

—Robert Malone, MD, MA

I believe that exercising our *medical liberty* represents not only huge benefits for the rest of our lives, but as a nation, it could also be the beginning of a delicate grace to save our country from decades of government overreach.

No reasonable excuse exists for not making this breakthrough available to every American. These are not the foundational days of hormone replacement with needles and creams with scary side effects. This is holistic and all natural and should be a birthright for every American as we age.

Here is an up-to-the-minute study: I have used bioidentical hormone replacement pellets for over ten years, restoring optimal hormone levels to thousands of patients of all ages, men and women, with no major complications and the highest patient satisfaction I have ever seen.

That brings up the whole issue of *medical freedom*. I want the *medical freedom* to respond to my patients' needs without government or insurance interference. I have done that. Insurance companies do not dictate the medicine I can practice. You want to be able to choose your care. That comes with a responsibility to educate yourself by choosing whatever provider or procedure you think will be in the best interests of your health without the health bureaucracy muscling in on your decision.

My *medical liberty* and my patients' liberty stays top-of-mind for me in everything I do. We have become (at the moment) perhaps the only clinical service in the nation that only uses bioidentical hormone pellets, gently inserted beneath the skin, to provide steady hormone replacement for months. After caring for thousands of men and women with this life-changing innovation, we have learned that there is no comparison—anywhere.

TIMELINE OF BIOIDENTICAL HORMONE REPLACEMENT IN AMERICA

1902

The English physician E. H. Starling discovered the first hormone, secretin, in collaboration with the physiologist W. M. Bayliss.

1935

Pellets were first used in women.

Bioidentical hormones were first used for menopausal symptom relief in the 1930s, after Canadian researcher James Collip developed a method to extract an orally active estrogen from the urine of pregnant women and marketed it as the active agent in a product called Emmenin.

1937

Pellets were first used in men.

1930s and 1940s

Estrogen replacement therapy was marketed to women by major pharmaceutical companies.[94]

1980s

In the late 1980s, the micronization of bioidentical steroids allowed the absorption of progesterone orally and estradiol, estriol, and testosterone in therapeutic amounts via transdermal routes.

1980–2000

Hormone replacement therapy (HRT) in the United States enjoyed a place of privilege and popularity throughout the 1980s and '90s, reaching its peak in 1999 with more than 85 million prescriptions written for women in that year alone.

2006

In October 2006, a controversial new book was published by Suzanne Somers, an avid proponent of bioidentical hormones.

2008

Abraham Morgentaler, MD, published the landmark book *Testosterone for Life* (McGraw-Hill, 2008).

2019

I helped redesign a custom-designed bioidentical pellet for easier, more comfortable insertion. Our new pellet was designed in more of a cylinder with rounded edges than previous tiny football-shaped pellets. And they were 99.5 percent either 17-beta testosterone or estradiol, the estrogen. The other 0.5 percent was a binding agent using natural fat.

2020

I published *The Hormone Handbook*.

2022

I began writing *Restore*.

This has become just too good and important to our culture to allow this holistic breakthrough to be clinically managed by insurance executives. We have allowed them to create a massive bureaucracy populated by surely well-meaning people who should have no business telling physicians what to do, when, and how to do it. Our new bioidentical hormone replacement practice lets nothing get between the physician and the patient. I believe that in the coming years, more and more people will push back on the broken medical system and that *medical liberty* just may be what ultimately bonds us again.

And because I have not brought this into the world of insurance, we have been able to advance the pellet and placement technology at a rapid pace. We lowered our fees. A year of hormone replacement and monitoring hormone levels now averages around $4 to $7 a day, not counting the periodic blood tests. Instead of charging for every visit, I set a one-time modest fee *for life* for your consults.

When a physician accepts insurance, that can be the end of proper medicine. They tell you how to practice, what procedures you will be allowed to do, what pharmaceuticals to use, and when and how often you can have this based on their algorithms, profit picture, policy language, and what the pharmaceutical companies permit.

The scorekeepers of our culture have fallen asleep on their watch. Our government has gotten too big and so busy managing every part of our lives that it has run a red light.

Here is something that can vastly improve the health and quality of aging of everyone with almost no side effects. What a fantastic effect this could have on people realizing the inevitable downside of aging.

> **Here is something that can vastly improve the health and quality of aging of everyone with almost no side effects. What a fantastic effect this could have on people realizing the inevitable downside of aging.**

As a nation with advanced medical capabilities, we need to stop thinking of sick care, and we need to finally start thinking about preventive wellness.

Going again to my metaphor of the car—you take your car in every five thousand miles to change the oil, rotate the tires, and change the air filter so that the transmission and the engine do not break. In medicine today, it's just the opposite. We wait for the symptoms to come, we become ill, and then we get the attention of the medical system. If we wait long enough, the engine breaks. If we had done our preventive maintenance, you would not be sitting in your dead car alongside the highway, scanning the horizon for the tow truck.

I would rather go preventive and optimize the beautiful bodies we've been given. This paradigm shift has been wished for by leading healthcare thinkers for decades. Well, now we can optimize our body and replace the hormones we have lost that lead to all this illness in the first place.

I think there's another shift there too. *Restore* is a verb, just like *live* is a verb.

Start thinking about choice and *medical freedom* and liberty. There are well-meaning people in the insurance field, but unfortunately, these companies have lost their way over time. Now a Communist mentality is at play within the modern healthcare system.

"Don't worry; we'll feed you. You're going to get enough food to eat, but it may be bread and water. You have no chance with us of steak and lobster."

And because this policy has become so expensive, many gratefully shuffle up to it and try to feel protected.

Back to my car analogy again. *We'll help pay for your gas*; that's what insurance covers. What the insurance should cover is the maintenance required to prevent your engine from exploding.

We have faceless bureaucrats dictating your care. That, to me, is anathema to liberty and choice for my body. We'll use diabetes as an example. Let's say there are four treatment options. They will select the option. You have that picked for you by someone you do not even know.

"Well, what if one of the other treatments works better?"

"Nope, we don't cover that. No can do."

Everything's an agreement with the company that does this plan. Everything's a backdoor deal dictated to us. I am tired of it. The king or queen of your health should be in your mirror. What happens to your body should definitely be your call. You decide. And that's my paradigm shift. The insurance companies should protect us from catastrophic events. And quit telling doctors how to practice medicine.

Frédéric Bastiat, the great French economist, statesman and journalist of the midnineteenth century, left a warning about this in his small but powerful book *The Law*, published in 1850.[95] Bastiat sailed the Atlantic to see what this great republic was like. What struck him most was the country's equality of conditions and its republic. Many scholars consider *The Law* as both the best written on the concept of a republic and the best written on America.

His observations of American independence left behind as clear a statement that has ever been made of the original ideal of American government as proclaimed in the Declaration of Independence, that any government's main purpose is to protect the lives, liberties, and properties of its citizens. These "three gifts from God precede all human legislation."[96]

"Life, liberty, and property do not exist because men have made laws. On the contrary, it was the fact that life, liberty, and property existed beforehand that caused men to make laws in the first place," he said.[97]

As he composed this little book in the 1840s, he was also alarmed at how the law had been perverted into what he called an "instrument of legal plunder."[98] Bastiat's warnings of the dire effects of legal plunder echo true today.

"Even when the government is a benevolent government, taking care of everyone's needs will lead to a society of complicated bureaucracy that oppresses innovation and individualism," he predicted.[99] As he warned, 172-plus years later, a labyrinth of arbitrary and capricious red tape awaits any meaningful scientific advancement like this phenomenal breakthrough.

The governmental medical interference with the smallest clinical detail takes your breath away.

I love liberty. But we have allowed our government to overextend its reach. It's gotten too big to control, resulting in a slowed pace of innovation and scientific breakthroughs in medicine. Our government has created alliances with the nation's insurance companies and pharmaceutical companies, and that alliance colors a determined quest for wealth and profits. Physicians have become numb to it. This keeps getting worse because not enough people have chirped about it, and business leaders will accept any way possible to lower their benefit costs.

"That cataract surgery recommended does not quite meet our requirements in size and shape in order to approve your surgery (even though the patient cannot drive at night due to glare); you may ask permission again next year."

"We'll approve your hormone pellets if they are synthetic. We're not sure yet about bioidentical hormone replacement. You're on your own."

"We will not approve payment for this because a compound pharmacy prepared it, not a giant international corporate manufacturer."

We need to work on this. Well-meaning bureaucratic folks often do not operate with the patient's best interests in mind. It seems like they have had their empathy surgically removed, coldly directing physicians in how to care for their patients, even though board-certified doctors have over thirty thousand hours of intensive training. People with chronic pain or disease do not get their medicine, while insurance providers argue with the doctor about finding a lower-cost choice that fits into their business plan. They incent us not to get care, even when we need it, with penalizing monthly fees, copays, deductibles, and drug tiers, which form the basis of their business model: a government-approved, heartless, soulless, on-off switch when the essential gets expensive.

That sounds harsh. But maybe well earned. That's what you get when you create a process that was supposed to help people but take your eye off the ball. At the same time, it evolves into a heartless, faceless, paternalistic mass of regulations that disappoints everyone it touches. Founders of our nation warned us about the government growing out of control.

WAITING FOR THE GOVERNMENT TO SAY IT'S OK

And if you don't pay attention, I fear you will miss the bus. If you wait for the government to say it's OK, the average time such breakthroughs get to the consumer is 16.5 years.[100]

Biomedical scientists have long felt the tension between their desire to perform innovative clinical research and the bureaucratic red tape that aims to protect patients. For years, scientists have been complaining about the rules and regulations that can hold up the progression of their biomedical research from the bench to the bedside.

A major study highlighted this problem. The authors examined thirty-two scientific papers describing effective medical interventions, each with more than one thousand citations, which, they argue, suggests that the publications represent scientific milestones."[101]

"Within the scope of the study, the average 'translational lag'— the time between a discovery and the first highly cited study showing its clinical usefulness—was 16.5 years, with a range of 0–221 years."[102]

All modern medicine moves incrementally forward. Does the discovery of a cure or remedy happen in an instant? No. It's hundreds, thousands of dedicated scientists putting together ideas, trying new things, and gathering evidence. Until the bureaucrats get a hold of it, then you can kick back, raise your kids, get them through school, and by then, maybe this will be okey-dokied by our government if the insurance companies and pharmaceutical companies don't get in the way.

Meanwhile, the two decades of wonderful rejuvenation and quality of life you could have experienced pass you by.

> *We do not become conscious of the three greatest blessings*
> *in life, such as health, youth, and freedom, as long as*
> *we possess them, but only after we've lost them.*

—ARTHUR SCHOPENHAUER (1788-1816)

Time does not pause. We are all getting older every day. The time to intervene in what makes us grow too old, too quickly, has come. Do not wait for the government to bless every aspect of bioidentical hormone replacement therapy—they can't and won't anytime soon. Why not? Because it's not in their best interest. If you wait, you'll miss this opportunity to discover your youthful wellness again.

We have proven that we can perform this medical practice without any connection with insurance, eliminate unneeded inter-mediaries, and significantly lower costs while creating an atmosphere of excellence in medicine without interference. I have been successful for over a decade practicing medicine the way I have been trained. Nothing stands between my patient and me, educating them, giving them options for their care, and offering choices.

People are weary of the government getting between them and their trusted healers. I hope we are nearing the day when *medical liberty* will be the issue that unites us as a nation, regardless of party affiliation. I sense great support from everyone I meet, and the power of the new availability of youthful aging, now a legitimate choice, will soon become more potent than our desire to be controlled. The paternalistic attitude of our national healthcare "brain trust" needs to be beached like a rusty submarine.

Bastiat offered much wisdom in *The Law*, much of which holds today. This closing thought in his book brings illuminates the problem:

> *I cannot avoid coming to this conclusion—that there are too many great men (and women) in the world … There are too many legislators, organizers, institutors of society, conductors of the people, fathers of nations, etc., etc. Too many persons place themselves above mankind, to rule and patronize it; too many persons make a trade of looking after it … and if I join the reformers, it is solely for the purpose of inducing them to relax their hold."[103]*

—FRÉDÉRIC BASTIAT (1801–1850)

What can you do? You can win your personal battle. It would be best if you had your health at peak levels to go up against imperious bureaucrats, the technocratic elites, or gate-crash the parties of middlemen getting between you and your trusted healers. Get your youthful wellness renewal done. Sleep well, eat well, and restore your hormones. *Boom.* Then pursue your dreams. Stand up for your liberty. Live your life like a free person. Pursue it politely, with civility. Don't be told *no*. I want people to understand that we all can aspire to be a lion, not a sheep. You can't be a lion if you're hungry. You can't be a lion if you're weak. Predators come for the weak.

Occasionally, a patient will come in and say, "Greg, I hope insurance will pay for this one day."

And I reply, "Sure. They may one day, but they'll tell you what dose, what medium (pill, salve, injection, pellet) route, the brand of the pellets, and how much you can have, all based on the lower bidder. They're going to say maybe the shots are better because they're cheaper. But they're not better long term. They may say the creams are better because their choice of manufacturer paid a lobbyist to go to the insurance company to get on a formulary. Are you ready to give up this free choice? Be careful what you ask for. Liberty is a choice. It's a verb."

I urge everyone to *choose wisely*. Choose a path taking advantage of new science to make our remaining years full of life and energy, or to watch our wellness dissipate, and in so doing, miss the most significant opportunity in our lifetime to begin to age gracefully.

This may represent the first choice you face, to choose to do a hormone replacement or not, and I pray you *do not choose poorly*. That would be to ignore the evidence and wait for guidance from people who have no idea what they are doing. Study the science.

Restore gives you all the tools you need. What is not provided in this important message is your own view of your life. Choose wisely, not based on what government or insurance executives say you may do, but on what you and your *trusted healer* decide to do. Now that this powerful renewal of your body has become a choice you can make, here and now, we finally can say: *Here's the science. Make your call.*

It's time we, as a nation, gave medicine back to the doctors. As our government incessantly drives a wedge between a healer and a patient, we need to express our *medical liberty*. Perhaps one day, we can all say politely, "No, thank you." Please notice that I use the term, "our government." It's ours, not theirs. They never told you this; not being tuned into alternative options for your health is just not your fault. It's just that until the last few years, much misinformation has confused people, mostly from our own government, unfortunately.

But today, we are taking the power back into our own hands. So let's take a close look under the hood and expand your knowledge of these alternative energy sources for your body through the miraculous power of bioidentical hormone replacement treatment.

SCIENCE AND COMMUNICATION, AND HOW RANGES AND VALUES ARE CREATED

I would come in armed with only curiosity, and my own natural ignorance. I was learning the value of bringing my ignorance to the surface … Ignorance was my ally, as long as it was backed up by curiosity. Ignorance without curiosity is not so good, but with curiosity, it was the clear water through which I could see the coins at the bottom of the fountain.[104]

—ALAN ALDA, IF I UNDERSTOOD YOU, WOULD I HAVE THIS LOOK ON MY FACE?

Best known for playing Hawkeye Pierce on the TV series *M*A*S*H,* Alan Alda is also a film and theater actor, scriptwriter, director, nonfiction author, science-show host, and founder of two organizations designed to help people improve their communication skills—a topic he covers in his new book *If I Understood You, Would I Have This Look on My Face?*

With deep respect for Mr. Alda, that's what I have been trying to do with you and me, exploring the new world of replacing your depleted hormones. Like Alan Alda, you got here because of your curiosity, and I hold Mr. Alda in great respect, especially because we scientists need all the help we can get with communications.

"Well," he told *Harvard Business Review* writer Alison Beard in 2017, "I'd always been interested in science, and when I was asked to do *Scientific American Frontiers* on *PBS*, I said I would if I could interview the people, not just read a narration, because I wanted to learn. The way we did that show was unusual. I didn't go in with a set of questions. I just went in with my curiosity, and my goal was to get them to explain their work to me in a way that

I could understand it, so that the audience would have a better understanding of it too."[105]

In the same interview, Alda admitted to trying to cultivate his own curiosity:

> I hope to cultivate it by, for example, helping scientists be open about their own curiosity. Often when they talk to the public about their work, it's a story told backwards. They tell you the end result, but they don't tell you what prompted them to search for it. They don't tell you what the obstacles were, the disasters that occurred, the wrong turns they took in getting to their final discovery. That's where the drama is. That's where we realize that science is a human experience. These people aren't gods. They're not secret masters of the universe. They have the same way of working things out that we do.[106]

So our story has encountered some drama, wrong turns, disasters, and ultimately, our final discoveries.

And when I take exception to the way laboratory ranges are developed or how out of date they may be, I am expressing the results of my curiosity and asking my colleagues to develop the same "question everything" mentality—kind of like Hawkeye in *M*A*S*H*.

One of the most important tools in all of medicine is "reference intervals" or "normal values" provided by our laboratories as they test our bodily fluids to help diagnose illness.

My own curiosity has led me to seek alternatives for these "ranges." The reference intervals in American medicine today are mystifying. Normal value ranges may vary among different laboratories. Some labs use different measurements or test different samples. Some ranges are endorsed by medical societies such as the Endocrine Society or the Institute of Medicine.

Selecting an optimal range for you may vary from the published values. Yet these ranges are essential. They can show changes over time and trends. I applaud using the term "reference interval" instead of "normal range." We use this information not for a diagnosis per se but for reference.

Here's a great example. Our population has seen a steady decrease in male testosterone levels over the past twenty years. Why? We believe this trend has been caused by increasingly compromised health and environmental factors. Sperm count measurements are also dwindling all over the globe. In 1992, a *British Medical Journal* study found a global 50 percent decline in sperm counts in men over the previous sixty years.[107] Multiple studies over the years confirmed that initial finding, including a 2017 paper showing a 50–60 percent decline in sperm concentration between 1973 and 2011 in men from around the world.[108] That will not end well if it continues.

Both men and women have testosterone. However, levels are naturally higher in men. Low testosterone, or male hypogonadism, also called low T, describes a condition where your testicles don't produce enough testosterone. The Cleveland Clinic suggests that a low testosterone count (as measured in your blood) for adults is generally considered anything below 250 nanograms per deciliter (ng/dl).[109]

The American Urology Association sets the bar a bit higher at 300 ng/dl.[110] I recommend 900–1,300 ng/dl for men and 70–250 ng/dl for women.

So are average testosterone levels now considered low? The Cleveland Clinic says it's normal for testosterone levels to decline as people age. The average drops about 1 percent per year after age 30.[111]

An article entitled "A population-level decline in serum testosterone levels in American men," issued by the *Journal of Clinical Endocrinology and Metabolism* in 2007, sounded the alarm. The numbers are getting worse.[112]

"These results indicate that recent years have seen a substantial, as yet unrecognized, age-independent population-level decrease in T in American men, potentially attributable to birth cohort differences or health or environmental effects not captured in observed data."[113]

"We're consistently seeing testosterone levels lower than we'd expect because of excessive weight and related health conditions—and that is alarming from a long-term perspective," says Cleveland Clinic endocrinologist Kevin Pantalone, DO.[114]

A Population-Level Decline in Serum Testosterone Levels in American Men

Total and calculated bioavailable T concentrations, by study wave and corresponding age range				TT (ng/dl)[a]		Bioavailable T (ng/dl)[a]	
Study wave	Study wave	Age range (yr)	n	Median	Interquartile range	Median	Interquartile range
T1	1987-89	45-71	1383	501	392-614	237	179-294
T2	1995-97	50-80	955	435	350-537	188	150-234
T3	2002-04	57-80	568	391	310-507	130	101-163

[a] May be converted to nmol/liter via multiplication by 0.03467.

T.G. Travison, A.B. Araujo, A.B. O'Donnell, V. Kupelian, J.B. McKinlay, Journal of Clinical Endocrinology and Metabolism, "A population-level decline in serum testosterone levels in American men." https://pubmed.ncbi.nlm.nih.gov/17062768/, January 2007, accessed January 15, 2023.

But while there's a downward trend in age-specific testosterone levels, averages haven't fallen to the point where they're in the "low" range for the overall population. But they are edging closer year by year.

There are no optimal numbers. All these ranges are based on averages of those citizens tested, and our citizens are not well. We base our ranges on what we see as optimal or what it would be if there were no endocrine disruptors (plastics, statins, obesity, sedentary lifestyle, etc.) if people were at a healthy weight and had a healthy diet and lifestyle. Reference ranges can differ between laboratories due to varying operating conditions, differing criteria for selecting healthy subjects, and different populations. Test results can be confusing.

So, what's optimal is, to try to go back to before pollution disrupted our bodies, what I call the "pre–neuroendocrine disruptor era." I want to go back as far as we can find data. What was the range then? Can we look at military records, hospital records, anything to help us find that moment before everything went haywire with our environment? Because that will represent a normal value, a normal reference range. And it becomes a target for optimal levels of hormones.

Literally, just five years ago, 1,200 was considered high normal. When I was in school, it was roughly 800 to 1,400.

But with the high end, there is no detriment to having too much testosterone. If a guy came into a urologist office with his level at 1,600, what's the treatment to lower it? None. The body will excrete what it does not need. Do any of these labs take that into account?

Therefore, speak to your physician about anything you don't understand or are concerned about.

The Centers for Disease Control (CDC) says that 70 percent of today's medical decisions depend on laboratory test results, showing the critical role of clinical laboratories in today's healthcare system. There are about 260,000 CLIA-certified laboratories (Clinical Laboratory Improvement Amendments) across the country, representing the cornerstone of diagnostic medicine today, which performs 14 billion laboratory tests annually.[115]

For diabetes, we shoot for an optimal number. We know optimal fasting blood sugar is between 70 and 80. We would not settle for 130. Never. We would not settle for a number based on age. We know this can lead to a heart attack or stroke.

111

Looking back everywhere we can, we research studies of healthy people because most studies on low T, even back in the 1930s and 1940s, are in a compromised population. What was our average soldier's score? What was our regular guy or gal, the average eighteen-to-twenty-five-year-old doing solid pull-ups, push-ups, and running?

We do not have a widely accepted placebo group untainted by aluminum, mercury vaccines, polyglycol, Roundup, and atrazine. We are bombarded. As a clinical goal, we try to restore the values in the preplastic, prepetroleum era, as far back as we can go, because that's more of an optimal range when our testicles and ovaries were not influenced by the outside toxins as much as today.

AGING EFFECT ON LABORATORY VALUES

Common is not normal, right? If something's common, that does not make it normal; there's either an optimal number or there isn't. I never want to hear, *It's common for your age.* Most importantly, you need to have a baseline hormone panel. Even if the ranges are skewed or debatable among clinicians, the trending matters the most.

Organ function declines with age and correlates with changes in laboratory values. Understanding the effect of age on laboratory values can increase diagnostic accuracy.

For example, according to ClinLab Navigator:

- Cholesterol increases by 30–40 mg/dL by age sixty.

- Creatinine clearance decreases by 10 mL/min/1.73 m2 per decade. Serum creatinine may not change noticeably due to decreasing muscle mass.

- HDL cholesterol decreases by 30 percent in postmenopausal women.

- Hemoglobin and hematocrit decrease slightly if at all, so low levels should not be attributed to aging.

- Magnesium decreases by 15 percent.

- PSA levels up to 6.5 ng/mL may be expected in men over 70.

- Postprandial glucose increases 30–40 mg/dL per decade after age forty. Fasting glucose changes minimally. Free testosterone decreases in men with age.[116]

To illustrate the importance of trending, if (as a man) you had a score of 265 ng/dl for your testosterone today (and if on this day the Labcorp reference interval is 264–916),[117] how does that compare with your baseline panel? What's the trend over time? Everybody needs this baseline.

That's why we treat symptoms, never numbers.

There are certain diseases for which you treat numbers (diabetes, of course).

There are clinical situations where the blood chemistry is predictably out of the reference interval. In pregnancy, when white blood cells are in the bloodstream, they also adhere to the lining. They can uncouple from the lining, resulting in a higher white count because they have departed the lining. It's not indicating a disease; they've moved. A woman with a white count of 13,000, pregnant with no symptoms, is expected then.

We use ranges as an *indicator*. Equally important, we listen to the patient. We trust the patient; they know their body more than we do. Who else knows? Their spouse. How our patients feel and what symptoms they may be having tells us a lot. It's a key measure for bioidentical hormone replacement therapy. Sure, we observe the numbers, but we also listen carefully to how the patient responds to the renewal of youthful chemistry. Then we can react with diet or additional hormones if we can do something to help with any minor side effects. The Optimal Bio team has assembled and tallied patient satisfaction scores for the last twenty years. We have an extraordinary patient satisfaction rate among our twenty thousand patients.

The *Canadian Medical Association Journal* published an article in 2020 entitled, "What Happens When Laboratory Reference Ranges Change?" The journal noted that although clinicians understand the importance of reference ranges to the interpretation of laboratory results and use them in daily practice, "few concern themselves with how such ranges are constructed. They may believe that these ranges have been rigorously established and are therefore always robust."[118]

Author Duncan J. Topliss, MD, added that clinical biochemists indeed "take great care in providing ranges that are as robust as possible, but there are substantial difficulties in establishing reliable reference ranges. Construction of reference ranges requires sufficient numbers of healthy individuals distributed over the range of ages and genders."[119]

"When constructing reference ranges, it's also important to define who is 'healthy' and to consider the importance of subclinical disease states," Dr. Topliss suggested.[120]

That underscores the fact that we have a sick population, and we're just not sure what disease states are affecting our testing population, but we are sure it affects the results. What's missing is a placebo population. Where would we find a perfectly healthy control group? It does not exist.

> I looked back at some patient charts in my office. On June 30, 2017, the testosterone range was listed as 348 to 1,197. And the very next day, July 1, 2017, it was changed to 264 to 916. Pretty big difference, all based on what Labcorp was seeing at the time.

Pre-Pellet Labs - Male

Patient ID:
Specimen ID:

DOB:
Age: **30**

Ordering Physician:

● labcorp

Lipid Panel w/ Chol/HDL Ratio (Cont.)
Lipid Panel w/ Chol/HDL Ratio

	Men	Women
1/2 Avg.Risk	3.4	3.3
Avg.Risk	5.0	4.4
2X Avg.Risk	9.6	7.1
3X Avg.Risk	23.4	11.0

Hepatic Function Panel (7)

Test	Current Result and Flag	Previous Result and Date	Units	Reference Interval
Protein, Total [01]	6.7		g/dL	6.0-8.5
Albumin [01]	4.7		g/dL	4.1-5.2
Bilirubin, Total [01]	0.4		mg/dL	0.0-1.2
Bilirubin, Direct [01]	0.12		mg/dL	0.00-0.40
Alkaline Phosphatase [01]	70		IU/L	44-121
	Please note reference interval change			
AST (SGOT) [01]	23		IU/L	0-40
ALT (SGPT) [01]	18		IU/L	0-44

Testosterone, Free and Total

Test	Current Result and Flag	Previous Result and Date	Units	Reference Interval
Testosterone [01]	289		ng/dL	264-916
	Adult male reference interval is based on a population of healthy nonobese males (BMI <30) between 19 and 39 years old. Travison, et.al. JCEM 2017,102;1161-1173. PMID: 28324103.			
Free Testosterone(Direct) [01]	9.9		pg/mL	8.7-25.1

Luteinizing Hormone(LH)

Test	Current Result and Flag	Previous Result and Date	Units	Reference Interval
LH [01]	2.6		mIU/mL	1.7-8.6

Prostate-Specific Ag

Test	Current Result and Flag	Previous Result and Date	Units	Reference Interval
Prostate Specific Ag [01]	0.8		ng/mL	0.0-4.0
	Roche ECLIA methodology. According to the American Urological Association, Serum PSA should decrease and remain at undetectable levels after radical prostatectomy. The AUA defines biochemical recurrence as an initial PSA value 0.2 ng/mL or greater followed by a subsequent confirmatory PSA value 0.2 ng/mL or greater. Values obtained with different assay methods or kits cannot be used interchangeably. Results cannot be interpreted as absolute evidence of the presence or absence of malignant disease.			

Estradiol

Test	Current Result and Flag	Previous Result and Date	Units	Reference Interval
Estradiol [01]	12.4		pg/mL	7.6-42.6
	Roche ECLIA methodology			

labcorp

Date Created and Stored 10/21/21 0542 ET **Final Report** Page 2 of 4

Sample bloodwork scores from Optimal Bio

Pre-Pellet Labs - Female

Hepatic Function Panel (7)

Test	Current Result and Flag	Previous Result and Date	Units	Reference Interval
Protein, Total [01]	7.1		g/dL	6.0-8.5
Albumin [01]	4.4		g/dL	3.8-4.9
Bilirubin, Total [01]	0.3		mg/dL	0.0-1.2
Bilirubin, Direct [01]	<0.10		mg/dL	0.00-0.40
Alkaline Phosphatase [01]	118		IU/L	44-121
AST (SGOT) [01]	26		IU/L	0-40
ALT (SGPT) [01]	16		IU/L	0-32

Testosterone, Free and Total

Test	Current Result and Flag	Previous Result and Date	Units	Reference Interval
Testosterone [01]	11		ng/dL	4-50
Free Testosterone (Direct) [01]	1.5		pg/mL	0.0-4.2

Luteinizing Hormone (LH)

Test	Current Result and Flag	Previous Result and Date	Units	Reference Interval
LH [01]	41.4		mIU/mL	

```
Adult Female:
   Follicular phase      2.4 -   12.6
   Ovulation phase      14.0 -   95.6
   Luteal phase          1.0 -   11.4
   Postmenopausal        7.7 -   58.5
```

FSH

Test	Current Result and Flag	Previous Result and Date	Units	Reference Interval
FSH [01]	97.8		mIU/mL	

```
Adult Female:
   Follicular phase      3.5 -   12.5
   Ovulation phase       4.7 -   21.5
   Luteal phase          1.7 -    7.7
   Postmenopausal       25.8 -  134.8
```

Prolactin

Test	Current Result and Flag	Previous Result and Date	Units	Reference Interval
Prolactin [01]	10.6		ng/mL	4.8-23.3

Estradiol

Test	Current Result and Flag	Previous Result and Date	Units	Reference Interval
Estradiol [01]	7.2		pg/mL	

```
Adult Female:
   Follicular phase     12.5 -   166.0
   Ovulation phase      85.8 -   498.0
   Luteal phase         43.8 -   211.0
   Postmenopausal       <6.0 -    54.7
Pregnancy
   1st trimester       215.0 - >4300.0
```

Roche ECLIA methodology

Sample bloodwork scores from Optimal Bio

In 2019, finally, clinicians began calling for testosterone therapy for women. There are no clearly established indications for testosterone therapy for females. Nonetheless, clinicians have treated women with testosterone for decades, with the intention of alleviating a variety of symptoms, with uncertain benefits and risks.

As crucial as testosterone is for women as well as men, try to find a consensus reference interval for females. Many women have never even had a testosterone blood test.

The "Global Consensus Position Statement on the Use of Testosterone Therapy for Women" noted that in most countries, physicians prescribe testosterone therapy "off-label" (or not typically prescribed) such that women are using either testosterone formulations approved for men, with dose modification or compounded therapies. Because of these issues, they have built a compelling case for a global consensus position statement on testosterone therapy for women based on the available evidence from placebo/comparator randomized controlled trials (RCTs).[121]

The character played by Alda in *M*A*S*H* is Hawkeye. After his medical residency in Boston, Hawkeye is drafted into the US Army Medical Corps and called to serve at the 4077th Mobile Army Surgical Hospital (M*A*S*H) during the Korean War. PBS's Dr. Howard Markel writes that "between long, intense sessions of treating critically wounded patients, he makes the best of his life in an isolated army camp with heavy drinking, carousing, and pulling pranks on the people around him, especially the unpleasantly stiff and callous Major Frank Burns and Major Margaret 'Hot Lips' Houlihan."[122]

LISTENING

In the 2018 interview by *The New Yorker* writer Howard Fishman, Alan Alda, now in his eighties, expressed his love of listening. "The question is academic," Fishman noted. "Alda's Hawkeye became (and remains) one of the most famous characters in television history. Like Alda himself, his Hawkeye is kind, articulate, and caring. In the show, Alda reacts as much as he acts. One of his greatest gifts as a performer is how well he seems to listen; a skill he says he learned early on in his career in improvisation class. 'The secret to good listening is simple,'" he told Fishman. "Unless I'm willing to be changed by you, I'm not really listening."[123]

Our government, which could, in a single graceful motion, make this available to millions of people, has not disapproved of bioidentical therapy, but it hasn't approved it either.

Our government is too big to listen to the people on the front lines. The FDA's two reports on BHRT in sixteen or so years indicate that the agency stopped listening years ago. Instead of tracking a breakthrough in clinical excellence, they can't seem to get away from making financially motivated clinical judgments for the physicians. The pharmaceutical and insurance corporations are not listening either. We need to listen for ourselves and quit waiting for the government to tell us what to do. Medical freedom lives.

A Special Reference
Provided by the
National Institutes of Health

The Miracle of Our Hormones[124]

T he hormones of the human body are very complex. They interact and guide your health. The National Institutes of Health shares this hormone educational material, which I include to make a point. Your hormone restoration will affect much more than your sex life.

Thanks to the National Library of Medicine, the National Center for Biotechnology Information for Open Access to the SEER Training modules, and the authors Suzanne Hiller-Sturmhofel, PhD, and Andrzej Bartke, PhD.

A plethora of hormones regulates many of the body's functions, including growth and development, metabolism, electrolyte balances, and reproduction. Numerous glands throughout the body produce hormones.

The hypothalamus produces several releasing and inhibiting hormones that act on the pituitary gland, stimulating the release of pituitary hormones. Of the pituitary hormones, several act on other glands located in various regions of the body, whereas other pituitary hormones directly affect their target organs.

Other hormone-producing glands throughout the body include the adrenal glands, which primarily produce cortisol; the gonads (i.e., ovaries and testes), which produce sex hormones; the thyroid, which produces thyroid hormone; the parathyroid, which produces parathyroid hormone; and the pancreas, which produces insulin and glucagon. Many of these hormones are part of regulatory hormonal cascades involving a hypothalamic hormone, one or more pituitary hormones, and one or more target gland hormones.

For the body to function properly, its various parts and organs must communicate with each other to ensure that a constant internal environment (i.e., homeostasis) is maintained. For example, neither the body temperature nor the levels of salts and minerals (i.e., electrolytes) in the blood must fluctuate beyond preset limits. Communication among various regions of the body also is essential for enabling the organism to respond appropriately to any changes in the internal and external environments.

Two systems help ensure communication: the nervous system and the hormonal (i.e., neuroendocrine) system. The nervous system generally allows rapid transmission (i.e., within fractions of seconds) of information between different body regions. Conversely, hormonal communication, which relies on the production and release of hormones from various glands and on the transport of those hormones via the bloodstream, is better suited for situations that require more widespread and longer-lasting regulatory actions. Thus, the two communication systems complement each other. In addition, both systems interact: stimuli from the nervous system can influence the release of certain hormones, and vice versa.

Hormones control the growth, development, and metabolism of the body; the electrolyte composition of bodily fluids; and reproduction. This article provides an overview of the hormone systems involved in those regulatory processes. The article first summarizes some of the basic characteristics of hormone-mediated communication within the body, then reviews the various glands involved in those processes and the major hormones they produce.

WHAT ARE HORMONES?

Hormones are molecules that are produced by endocrine glands, including the hypothalamus, pituitary gland, adrenal glands, gonads (i.e., testes and ovaries), thyroid gland, parathyroid glands, and pancreas. The term "endocrine" implies that in response to specific stimuli, the products of those glands are released into the bloodstream. The hormones then are carried via the blood to their target cells. Some hormones have only a few specific target cells, whereas other hormones affect numerous cell types throughout the body. The target cells for each hormone are characterized by the presence of certain docking molecules (i.e., receptors) for the hormone that are located either on the cell surface or inside the cell. The interaction between the hormone and its receptor triggers a cascade of biochemical reactions in the target cell that eventually modify the cell's function or activity.

Mechanisms of Action

Several classes of hormones exist, including steroids, amino acid derivatives, and polypeptides and proteins. Those hormone classes differ in their general molecular structures (e.g., size and chemical properties). As a result of the structural differences, their mechanisms of action (e.g., whether they can enter their target cells and how they modulate the activity of those cells) also differ. Steroids, which are produced by the gonads and part of the adrenal gland (i.e., the adrenal cortex), have a molecular structure like that of cholesterol. The molecules can enter their target cells and interact with receptors in the fluid that fills the cell (i.e., the cytoplasm) or in the cell nucleus. The hormone-receptor complexes then bind to certain regions of the cell's genetic material (i.e., the DNA), thereby regulating the activity of specific hormone-responsive genes.

Amino acid derivatives are modified versions of some of the building blocks of proteins. The thyroid gland and another region of the adrenal glands (i.e., the adrenal medulla) produce this type of hormone (i.e., the amino acid derivatives). Like steroids, amino acid derivatives can enter the cell, where they interact with receptor proteins that are already associated with specific DNA regions. The interaction modifies the activity of the affected genes.

Polypeptide and protein hormones are chains of amino acids of various lengths (from three to several hundred amino acids). These hormones are found primarily in the hypothalamus, pituitary gland, and pancreas. In some instances, they are derived from inactive pre-cursors, or prohormones, which can be cleaved into one or more active hormones. Because of their chemical structure, the polypeptide and protein hormones cannot enter cells. Instead, they interact with receptors on the cell surface. The interaction initiates biochemical changes in either the cell's membrane or interior, eventually modifying the cell's activity or function.

Regulation of Hormone Activity

To maintain the body's homeostasis and respond appropriately to changes in the environment, hormone production, and secretion must be tightly controlled. To achieve this control, many bodily functions are regulated not by a single hormone but by several hormones that regulate each other.

For example, for many hormone systems, the hypothalamus secretes so-called releasing hormones, which are transported via the blood to the pituitary gland. There, the releasing hormones induce the production and secretion of pituitary hormones, which in turn are transported by the blood to their target glands (e.g., the adrenal glands, gonads, or thyroid). In those glands, the interaction of the pituitary hormones with their respective target cells results in the release of the hormones that ultimately influence the organs targeted by the hormone cascade.

Constant feedback from the target glands to the hypothalamus and pituitary gland ensures that the activity of the hormone system involved remains within appropriate boundaries. Thus, in most cases, negative feedback mechanisms exist by which hormones released by the target glands affect the pituitary gland and/or hypothalamus. When certain predetermined blood levels of those hormones are reached, the hypothalamus and/or the pituitary cease hormone release, thereby turning off the cascade. In some instances, so-called short-loop feedback occurs, in which pituitary hormones directly act back on the hypothalamus.

The sensitivity with which these negative feedback systems operate (i.e., the target hormone levels that are required to turn off hypothalamic or pituitary hormone release) can change at different physiological states or stages of life. For example, the progressive reduction in sensitivity of the hypothalamus and pituitary to negative feedback by gonadal steroid hormones plays an important role in sexual maturation.

Although negative feedback is more common, some hormone systems are controlled by positive feedback mechanisms, in which a target gland hormone acts back on the hypothalamus and/or pituitary to increase the release of hormones that stimulate the secretion of the target gland hormone.

One such mechanism occurs during a woman's menstrual period: increasing estrogen levels in the blood temporarily stimulate, rather than inhibit, hormone release from the pituitary and hypothalamus, thereby further increasing estrogen levels and eventually leading to ovulation. Such a mechanism requires a specific threshold level, however, at which the positive feedback loop is turned off to maintain a stable system.

125

Hormones Produced by the Major Hormone-Producing (i.e., Endocrine) Glands and Their Primary Functions

ENDOCRINE GLAND	HORMONE	PRIMARY HORMONE FUNCTION
Hypothalamus	Corticotropin-releasing hormone (CRH)	Stimulates the pituitary to release adrenocortico-tropic hormone (ACTH)
	Gonadotropin-releasing hormone (GnRH)	Stimulates the pituitary to release luteinizing hormone (LH) and follicle-stimulating hormone (FSH)
	Thyrotropin-releasing hormone (TRH)	Stimulates the pituitary to release thyroid-stimulating hormone (TSH)
	Growth hormone-releasing hormone (GHRH)	Stimulates the release of growth hormone (GH) from the pituitary
	Somatostatin	Inhibits the release of GH from the pituitary
	Dopamine	Inhibits the release of prolactin from the pituitary
Anterior pituitary gland	ACTH	Stimulates the release of hormones from the adrenal cortex
	LH	In women, stimulates the production of sex hormones (i.e., estrogens) in the ovaries as well as during ovulation; in men, stimulates testosterone production in the testes

ENDOCRINE GLAND	HORMONE	PRIMARY HORMONE FUNCTION
	FSH	In women, stimulates follicle development; in men, stimulates sperm production
	TSH	Stimulates the release of thyroid hormone
	GH	Promotes the body's growth and development
	Prolactin	Controls milk production (i.e., lactation)
Posterior pituitary gland*	Vasopressin	Helps control the body's water and electrolyte levels
	Oxytocin	Promotes uterine contraction during labor and activates milk ejection in nursing women
Adrenal cortex	Cortisol	Helps control carbohydrate, protein, and lipid metabolism; protects against stress
	Aldosterone	Helps control the body's water and electrolyte regulation
Testes	Testosterone	Stimulates development of the male reproductive organs, sperm production, and protein anabolism

ENDOCRINE GLAND	HORMONE	PRIMARY HORMONE FUNCTION
Ovaries	Estrogen (produced by the follicle)	Stimulates development of the female reproductive organs
	Progesterone (produced by the corpus luteum)	Prepares uterus for pregnancy and mammary glands for lactation
Thyroid gland	Thyroid hormone (i.e., thyroxine [T4] and triiodo-thyronine [T3])	Controls metabolic processes in all cells
	Calcitonin	Helps control calcium metabolism (i.e., lowers calcium levels in the blood)
Parathyroid gland	Parathyroid hormone (PTH)	Helps control calcium metabolism (i.e., increases calcium levels in the blood)
Pancreas	Insulin	Helps control carbohydrate metabolism (i.e., lowers blood sugar levels)
	Glucagon	Helps control carbohydrate metabolism (i.e., increases blood sugar levels)

These hormones are produced in the hypothalamus but stored in and released from the posterior pituitary gland.

The Hypothalamus and Its Hormones

The hypothalamus is a small region located within the brain that controls many bodily functions, including eating and drinking, sexual functions and behaviors, blood pressure and heart rate, body temperature maintenance, the sleep-wake cycle, and emotional states (e.g., fear, pain, anger, and pleasure). Hypothalamic hormones play pivotal roles in the regulation of many of those functions.

Because the hypothalamus is part of the central nervous system, the hypothalamic hormones are produced by nerve cells (i.e., neurons). In addition, because signals from other neurons can modulate the release of hypothalamic hormones, the hypothalamus serves as the major link between the nervous and endocrine systems.

For example, the hypothalamus receives information from higher brain centers that respond to various environmental signals. Consequently, the hypothalamic function is influenced by both the external and internal environments as well as by hormone feedback. Stimuli from the external environment that indirectly influence hypothalamic function include the light-dark cycle; temperature; signals from other members of the same species; and a wide variety of visual, auditory, olfactory, and sensory stimuli.

The communication between other brain areas and the hypothalamus, which conveys information about the internal environment, involves electrochemical signal transmission through molecules called neurotransmitters (e.g., aspartate, dopamine, gamma-aminobutyric acid, glutamate, norepinephrine, and serotonin). The complex interplay of the actions of various neurotransmitters regulates the production and release of hormones from the hypothalamus.

The hypothalamic hormones are released into blood vessels that connect the hypothalamus and the pituitary gland (i.e., the hypothalamic-hypophyseal portal system). Because they generally promote or inhibit the release of hormones from the pituitary gland, hypothalamic hormones are commonly called releasing or inhibiting hormones.

Hypothalamic Hormones

- Corticotropin-releasing hormone (CRH)

- Regulates carbohydrate, protein, and fat metabolism as well as sodium and water balance in the body

- Gonadotropin-releasing hormone (GnRH)

- Controls sexual and reproductive functions, including pregnancy and lactation (i.e., milk production)

- Thyrotropin-releasing hormone (TRH)

- Controls the metabolic processes of all cells and which contributes to the hormonal regulation of lactation

- Growth hormone-releasing hormone (GHRH)

- Promoting the organism's growth (our bodies)

- Somatostatin

- Aids bone and muscle growth but has the opposite effect as that of GHRH

- Dopamine

- Functions primarily as a neurotransmitter but also has some hormonal effects, such as repressing lactation until it is needed after childbirth.

The Pituitary and Its Major Hormones

The pituitary (also sometimes called the hypophysis) is a gland about the size of a small marble located in the brain directly below the hypothalamus. The pituitary gland consists of two parts: the anterior pituitary and the posterior pituitary.

The Anterior Pituitary

The anterior pituitary produces several important hormones that either stimulate target glands (e.g., the adrenal glands, gonads, or thyroid gland) to produce target gland hormones or directly affect target organs. The pituitary hormones include adrenocorticotropic hormone (ACTH); gonadotropins; thyroid-stimulating hormone (TSH), also called thyrotropin; growth hormone (GH); and prolactin.

The first three of those hormones—ACTH, gonadotropins, and TSH—act on other glands. Thus, ACTH stimulates the adrenal cortex to produce corticosteroid hormones—primarily cortisol—as well as small amounts of female and male sex hormones. The gonadotropins comprise two molecules, luteinizing hormone (LH) and follicle-stimulating hormone (FSH).

These two hormones regulate the production of female and male sex hormones in the ovaries and testes as well as the production of the germ cells—that is, the egg cells (i.e., ova) and sperm cells (i.e., spermatozoa). TSH stimulates the thyroid gland to produce and release thyroid hormones. The remaining two pituitary hormones, GH and prolactin, directly affect their target organs.

Growth Hormones

Growth hormones (GHs) are the most abundant of the pituitary hormones. As the name implies, it plays a pivotal role in controlling the body's growth and development. For example, it stimulates the linear growth of the bones; promotes the growth of internal organs, fat (i.e., adipose) tissue, connective tissue, endocrine glands, and muscle; and controls the development of the reproductive organs. Accordingly, the GH levels in the blood are highest during early childhood and puberty and decline thereafter. Nevertheless, even relatively low GH levels still may be important later in life, and GH deficiency may contribute to some symptoms of aging.

In addition to its growth-promoting role, GH affects carbohydrate, protein, and fat (i.e., lipid) metabolism. Thus, GH increases the levels of sugar glucose in the blood by reducing glucose uptake by muscle cells and adipose tissue and by promoting glucose production (i.e., gluconeogenesis) from precursor molecules in the liver. (These actions are opposite to those of the hormone insulin.) GH also enhances the uptake of amino acids from the blood into cells, as well as their incorporation into proteins, and stimulates the breakdown of lipids in adipose tissue.

To elicit these various effects, GH modulates the activities of numerous target organs, including the liver, kidneys, bone, cartilage, skeletal muscle, and adipose cells. For some of these effects, GH acts directly on the target cells. In other cases, however, GH acts indirectly by stimulating the production of a molecule called insulinlike growth factor 1 (IGF-1) in the liver and kidneys. The blood then transports IGF-1 to the target organs, where it binds to specific receptors on the cells. This interaction then may lead to the increased DNA production and cell division that underlie the growth process.

Two hypothalamic hormones control GH release: (1) growth hormone-releasing hormone (GHRH), which stimulates GH release, and (2) somatostatin, which inhibits GH release. This regulatory mechanism also involves a short-loop feedback component, by which GH acts on the hypothalamus to stimulate somatostatin release. In addition, GH release is enhanced by stress, such as low blood sugar levels (i.e., hypoglycemia) or severe exercise, and by the onset of deep sleep.

Prolactin

Together with other hormones, prolactin plays a central role in the development of the female breast and in the initiation and maintenance of lactation after childbirth. Prolactin's function in men, however, is not well understood, although excessive prolactin release can lead to reduced sex drive (i.e., libido) and impotence. Several factors control prolactin release from the anterior pituitary. For example, prolactin is released in increasing amounts in response to the rise in estrogen levels in the blood that occurs during pregnancy. In nursing women, prolactin is released in response to suckling by the infant. Several releasing and inhibitory factors from the hypothalamus also control prolactin release. The most important of those factors is dopamine, which has an inhibitory effect.

The Posterior Pituitary

The posterior pituitary does not produce its own hormones; instead, it stores two hormones—vasopressin and oxytocin—that are produced by neurons in the hypothalamus. Both hormones collect at the ends of the neurons, which are in the hypothalamus and extend to the posterior pituitary.

Vasopressin, also called arginine vasopressin (AVP), plays an important role in the body's water and electrolyte economy. Thus, AVP release promotes the reabsorption of water from the urine in the kidneys. Through this mechanism, the body reduces urine volume and conserves water. AVP release from the pituitary is controlled by the concentration of sodium in the blood as well as by blood volume and blood pressure.

Oxytocin, the second hormone stored in the posterior pituitary, stimulates the contractions of the uterus during childbirth. In nursing women, the hormone activates milk ejection in response to suckling by the infant (i.e., the so-called letdown reflex).

The Adrenal Glands and Their Hormones

The adrenal glands are small structures located on top of the kidneys. Structurally, they consist of an outer layer (i.e., the cortex) and an inner layer (i.e., the medulla). The adrenal cortex produces numerous hormones, primarily corticosteroids (i.e., glucocorticoids and mineralocorticoids). The cortex is also the source of small amounts of sex hormones; those amounts, however, are insignificant compared with the amounts normally produced by the ovaries and testes. The adrenal medulla generates two substances—adrenaline and noradrenaline—that are released as part of the fight-or-flight response to various stress factors.

The primary glucocorticoid in humans is cortisol (also called hydro-cortisone), which helps control carbohydrate, protein, and lipid metabolism. For example, cortisol increases glucose levels in the blood by stimulating gluconeogenesis in the liver and promotes the formation of glycogen (i.e., a molecule that serves as the storage form of glucose) in the liver. Cortisol also reduces glucose uptake into muscle and adipose tissue, thereby opposing the effects of insulin. Furthermore, in various tissues, cortisol promotes protein and lipid breakdown into products (i.e., amino acids and glycerol, respectively) that can be used for gluconeogenesis.

In addition to those metabolic activities, cortisol appears to protect the body against the deleterious effects of various stress factors, including acute trauma, major surgery, severe infections, pain, blood loss, hypoglycemia, and emotional stress. All these stress factors lead to drastic increases in the cortisol levels in the blood. For people in whom cortisol levels cannot increase (e.g., because they had their adrenal glands removed), even mild stress can be fatal. Finally, high doses of cortisol and other corticosteroids can be used medically to suppress tissue inflammation in response to injuries and to reduce the immune response to foreign molecules.

The primary mineralocorticoid in humans is aldosterone, which also helps regulate the body's water and electrolyte balance. Its principal functions are to conserve sodium and to excrete potassium from the body. For example, aldosterone promotes the reabsorption of sodium in the kidney, thereby reducing water excretion and increasing blood volume. Similarly, aldosterone decreases the ratio of sodium to potassium concentrations in sweat and saliva, thereby preventing sodium loss via those routes. The effect can be highly beneficial in hot climates, where much sweating occurs.

In contrast to glucocorticoids, pituitary, or hypothalamic, hormones do not regulate aldosterone release. Instead, it is controlled primarily by another hormone system, the renin-angiotensin system, which also controls kidney function. In addition, the levels of sodium and potassium in the blood influence aldosterone levels.

The Gonads and Their Hormones

The gonads (i.e., the ovaries and testes) serve two major functions. First, they produce germ cells (i.e., ova in the ovaries and spermatozoa in the testes). Second, the gonads synthesize steroid sex hormones that are necessary for the development and function of both female and male reproductive organs and secondary sex characteristics (e.g., the adult distribution of body hair, such as facial hair in men) as well as for pregnancy, childbirth, and lactation.

Four types of sex hormones exist, each with different functions. In addition to reproductive functions, sex hormones play numerous essential roles throughout the body. For example, they affect the metabolism of carbohydrates and lipids, the cardiovascular system, and bone growth and development.

Estrogens

The major estrogen is estradiol, which, in addition to small amounts of estrone and estriol, is produced primarily in the ovaries. Other production sites of estrogens include the corpus luteum, the placenta, and the adrenal glands. In men and postmenopausal women, most estrogens present in the circulation are derived from the conversion of testicular, adrenal, and ovarian androgens. The conversion occurs in peripheral tissues, primarily adipose tissue, and skin.

The main role of estrogens is to coordinate the normal development and functioning of the female genitalia and breasts. During puberty, estrogens promote the growth of the uterus, breasts, and vagina; determine the pattern of fat deposition and distribution in the body that results in the typical female shape; regulate the pubertal growth spurt and cessation of growth at adult height; and control the development of secondary sexual characteristics. In adult women, the primary functions of estrogens include regulating the menstrual cycle, contributing to the hormonal regulation of pregnancy and lactation, and maintaining female libido.

During menopause, estrogen production in the ovaries ceases. The resulting reduction in estrogen levels leads to symptoms such as hot flashes, sweating, pounding of the heart (i.e., palpitations), increased irritability, anxiety, depression, and brittle bones (i.e., osteoporosis).

Progestogens

The ovaries produce progestogens during a certain phase of the menstrual cycle and in the placenta for most of pregnancy. Progestogens cause changes in the uterine lining in preparation for pregnancy and—together with estrogens—stimulate the development of the mammary glands in the breasts in preparation for lactation. The primary progestogen is progesterone.

Androgens

The principal androgenic steroid is testosterone, which is secreted primarily from the testes but also, in small amounts, from the adrenal glands (both in men and women) and from the ovaries. Its main function is to stimulate the development and growth of the male genital tract. In addition, testosterone has strong protein anabolic activities—that is, it promotes protein generation, which leads to increased muscle mass. The specific functions of testosterone vary during different developmental stages, as follows:

In the fetus, testosterone primarily ensures the development of the internal and external male genitalia.

During puberty, testosterone promotes the growth of the male sex organs and is responsible for other male developmental characteristics, such as the pubertal growth spurt and eventual cessation of growth at adult height; deepening of the voice; growth of facial, pubic, axillary, and body hair; and increase in muscularity and strength.

In the adult male, testosterone primarily serves to maintain masculinity, libido, and sexual potency as well as regulate sperm production. Testosterone levels decline slightly with age, although the drop is not as drastic as the reduction in estrogen levels in women during menopause.

The Thyroid and Its Hormones

The thyroid gland, which consists of two lobes, is in front of the windpipe (i.e., tracΩhea), just below the voice box (i.e., larynx). The gland produces two structurally related hormones, thyroxine (T4) and triiodothyronine (T3), which are iodinated derivatives of the amino acid tyrosine.

Both hormones are collectively referred to as "thyroid hormones." T4 constitutes approximately 90 percent of the hormone produced in the thyroid gland. However, T3 (10 percent) is a much more active hormone, and most of the T4 produced by the thyroid is converted into T3 in the liver and kidneys.[125]

Thyroid hormones in general serve to increase the metabolism of almost all body tissues. For example, the thyroid hormones stimulate the production of certain proteins involved in heat generation in the body, a function that is essential for maintaining body temperature in cold climates. Moreover, thyroid hormones promote several other metabolic processes involving carbohydrates, proteins, and lipids that help generate the energy required for the body's functions.

In addition to those metabolic effects, thyroid hormones play an essential role in the development of the central nervous system during late fetal and early postnatal developmental stages. Furthermore, thyroid hormones exert an effect similar to that of GH on normal bone growth and maturation. Finally, thyroid hormones are required for the normal development of teeth, skin, and hair follicles as well as for the functioning of the nervous, cardiovascular, and gastrointestinal systems.

In addition to the thyroid hormone, certain cells (i.e., parafollicular C cells) in the thyroid gland produce calcitonin, a hormone that helps maintain normal calcium levels in the blood. Specifically, calcitonin lowers calcium levels in the blood by reducing the release of calcium from the bones; inhibiting the constant erosion of bones (i.e., bone resorption), which also releases calcium; and inhibiting the reabsorption of calcium in the kidneys. Those effects are opposite to those of parathyroid hormone (PTH), which is discussed in the following section.

The Parathyroid Glands and Their Hormones

The parathyroid glands are four pea-sized bodies located behind the thyroid gland that produce parathyroid hormones (PTHs). These hormones increase calcium levels in the blood, helping to maintain bone quality and an adequate supply of calcium, which is needed for numerous functions throughout the body (e.g., muscle movement and signal transmission within cells). Specifically, PTHs cause the reabsorption of calcium from and excretion of phosphate in the urine. PTHs also promote the release of stored calcium from the bones as well as bone resorption, both of which increase calcium levels in the blood. Finally, PTHs stimulate the absorption of calcium from the food in the gastrointestinal tract. Consistent with PTHs's central role in calcium metabolism, the release of this hormone is not controlled by pituitary hormones but by the calcium levels in the blood. Thus, low calcium levels stimulate PTH release, whereas high calcium levels suppress it.

Many of the functions of PTHs require or are facilitated by a substance called 1,25-dihydroxycholecalciferol, a derivative of vitamin D. In addition, numerous other hormones are involved in regulating the body's calcium levels and bone metabolism, including estrogens, glucocorticoids, and growth hormone.

The Pancreas and Its Hormones

The pancreas is in the abdomen, behind the stomach, and serves two distinctly different functions. First, it acts as an exocrine organ, because the majority of pancreatic cells produce various digestive enzymes that are secreted into the gut, and which are essential for the effective digestion of food. Second, the pancreas serves as an endocrine organ, because certain cell clusters (i.e., the islets of Langerhans) produce two hormones—insulin and glucagon—that are released into the blood and play pivotal roles in blood glucose regulation.

Insulin

Insulin is produced in the beta cells of the islets of Langerhans. Its primary purpose is to lower blood glucose levels; in fact, insulin is the only blood sugar-lowering hormone in the body. To this end, insulin promotes the formation of storage forms of energy (e.g., glycogen, proteins, and lipids) and suppresses the breakdown of those stored nutrients. Accordingly, the target organs of insulin are primarily those that are specialized for energy storage, such as the liver, muscles, and adipose tissue. Specifically, insulin has the following metabolic effects:

- Promotes glucose uptake into cells and its conversion into glycogen, stimulates the breakdown of glucose, and inhibits gluconeogenesis

- Stimulates the transport of amino acids into cells and protein synthesis in muscle cells, thereby lowering the levels of amino acids available for gluconeogenesis in the liver

- Increases fat synthesis in the liver and adipose tissue, thereby lowering the levels of glycerol, which also can serve as a starting material for gluconeogenesis

The release of insulin is controlled by various factors, including blood glucose levels; other islet hormones (e.g., glucagon); and, indirectly, other hormones that alter blood glucose levels (e.g., GH, glucocorticoids, and thyroid hormone).

Glucagon

The second blood-sugar-regulating pancreatic hormone is glucagon, which is produced in the alpha cells of the islets of Langerhans.

Glucagon increases blood glucose levels; accordingly, its main actions generally are opposite to those of insulin. For example, glucagon increases glycogen breakdown and gluconeogenesis in the liver as well as the breakdown of lipids and proteins. The release of glucagon is regulated by many of the same factors as is insulin's release, but sometimes with the opposite effect. Thus, an increase in blood glucose levels stimulates insulin release but inhibits glucagon release.

A finely tuned balance between the activities of insulin and glucagon is essential for maintaining blood sugar levels. Accordingly, disturbances of that balance, such as an insulin deficiency or an inability of the body to respond adequately to insulin, result in serious disorders, such as diabetes mellitus. (For more information on diabetes and on alcohol's effects on insulin, glucagon, and the management of diabetes, see the article by Emanuele and colleagues, pages 211–219.)

Again, *applause for* the National Library of Medicine, the National Center for Biotechnology Information for Open Access to the SEER Training modules, and the authors Suzanne Hiller-Sturmhofel, PhD, and Andrzej Bartke, PhD.

Hormone Systems

As the reference article indicated in describing the various endocrine glands and their hormones, some hormones are controlled directly by the metabolic pathways that they influence.

For example, blood sugar levels directly control insulin and glucagon release by the pancreas, and calcium levels in the blood regulate PTH release.

Conversely, many hormones produced by target glands are regulated by pituitary hormones, which in turn are controlled by hypothalamic hormones. Examples of such regulatory hormonal cascades include the hypothalamic-pituitary-adrenal (HPA) axis, the hypothalamic-pituitary-gonadal (HPG) axis, and the hypothalamic-pituitary-thyroidal (HPT) axis.

The HPG Axis

In both men and women, the HPG axis is the hormone system that controls the release of sex hormones. In both genders, the system is activated by GnRH, which is released regularly in short bursts from the hypothalamus. GnRH then stimulates the release of FSH and LH from the anterior pituitary.

In men, LH stimulates certain cells in the testes (i.e., Leydig cells) to release testosterone. FSH and testosterone are key regulators of another set of testicular cells (i.e., Sertoli cells), which support and nourish the sperm cells during their maturation. The HPG axis in men is regulated through a variety of factors. For example, testosterone is part of a negative feedback mechanism that inhibits GnRH release by the hypothalamus and LH release by the pituitary. In addition, the Sertoli cells secrete a substance called inhibin, which prevents FSH release from the pituitary. Finally, the Leydig cells and, to a lesser extent, the Sertoli cells produce a substance called activin, which stimulates FSH secretion and thus has the opposite effects of inhibin.

In women, during the menstrual cycle, LH and FSH stimulate the ovarian follicle that contains the maturing egg to produce estradiol. After ovulation has occurred, LH also promotes production of progesterone and estradiol by the corpus luteum.

Both hormones participate in a negative feedback mechanism through most of the menstrual cycle, suppressing GnRH release from

143

the hypothalamus and LH release from the pituitary. Shortly before ovulation, however, a positive feedback mechanism is activated by which estradiol enhances LH release from the pituitary. The resulting surge in LH levels ultimately leads to ovulation, the formation of the corpus luteum, and progesterone release. Progesterone exerts negative feedback on LH and FSH release, causing LH levels to decline again. In addition to those mechanisms, FSH release from the pituitary is regulated by inhibin, a substance produced by certain cells in the ovarian follicle.

The HPT Axis

The hormones that make up the HPT axis control the metabolic processes of all cells in the body and are therefore crucial for the organism to function normally. The secretion of TRH from the hypothalamus activates the HPT axis. After reaching the pituitary, TRH stimulates the release of TSH, which in turn promotes the production and release of T4 and T3 by the thyroid gland. Negative feedback effects of T4 and T3 on both the hypothalamus and the pituitary regulate the HPT system.

SUMMARY

The neuroendocrine system is a highly complex and tightly controlled network of hormones released by endocrine glands throughout the body.

The levels of some of the hormones are regulated in a fairly straightforward manner by the end products that they influence.

Thus, blood sugar levels primarily regulate insulin and glucagon release by the pancreas. Other hormones (e.g., those of the HPA,

HPG, and HPT axes) are parts of hormone cascades whose activities are controlled through elaborate feedback mechanisms.

In addition, numerous indirect interactions exist between the various hormone systems governing body functioning. For example, hormones such as GH and thyroid hormone, through their effects on cellular metabolism, may modify blood sugar levels and, accordingly, insulin release.

5

Women's Lifetime of Choices for Optimal Health—It's Much More Than Estrogen

I have my hormones balanced. Most doctors give women synthetic hormones, which eliminate the symptoms, but it's doing nothing to replace the hormones you have lost. Without our hormones, we die.[126]

—SUZANNE SOMERS, AUTHOR OF

FOURTEEN *NEW YORK TIMES* BESTSELLERS

S uzanne Somers has authored over twenty books. Her most recent book release, *A New Way to Age: The Most Cutting-Edge Advances in Antiaging*, came out in January 2020, and it covers topics about aging well and natural alternatives that will increase your aging process to be a good one. Ms. Somers often says, "Hormones shape who we are."[127]

This thing called life is a thrilling adventure. It's mystical, spiritual, fulfilling, and constantly advancing. We have been given a gift, the human body. The constancy of the River of Time waits for no one. We all float downstream at the will of the water flow, but we are given an oar to steer us along, and we have choices along the way.

When I reflect on my three decades as an OB/GYN physician, I was honored to care for over fifty thousand women. I delivered approximately twelve thousand babies. I became a *trusted healer* for my patients. And I developed a deep appreciation for women's continuous, challenging journey.

Heck, men have it a lot easier. Our journey has been simpler. No less challenging—just more straightforward.

My goal is always to honor women and express my deep appreciation for their journey and every stage of that adventure. As I have said, we all grow old. We all die. But the physical changes in a woman are epic, continuous, and sometimes painful. Events come unbidden. Women bear the greatest gift of all, the ability to bring life into this world. Imagine being able to do that. It's a spiritual gift. Our Creator has given women the ability to create life.

The forces bearing down on women begin in puberty and adolescence, and stresses start to arrive: periods, sexuality, anxiety; then come the childbearing years, parenting stress, postpartum weight loss, postpartum blues, followed by midlife crisis, changing body shape and appearance with age, energy and stamina issues, mood swings, threats of heart disease, breast cancer, ovarian cancer, dementia, stroke, osteoporosis, then enduring hot flashes, menopause, perimenopause, postmenopause, thyroid hormone loss, sleep issues, libido issues, moods, brain fog, dealing with growing weakness, and all the while fighting off depression.

These symptoms are also a biological marker for endothelial dysfunction and scientists all over the world are looking at this as an area of interest, possibly being a part of the initiating process of atherosclerosis and dementia.

Whew.

Progesterone   Premarin   Estrogen

Progesterone Deficiency Symptoms	Estrogen Deficiency Symptoms
• Anxiety	• Anxiety
• Agitation	• Hot Flashes
• Breast Swelling/Tenderness	• Depression
• Bloating	• Decreased Libido
• Fluid Retention	• Difficulty Sleeping
• Headaches	• Headaches
• Mood Swings	• Decreased Memory
• Sleep Disturbances	• Fatigue
• Heavy or Irregular Menstrual Bleeding	• Dry Flaking Skin

And as we enter the final chapter of life, I still want even an eighty-five-year-old woman to be vibrant, strong of body, alert, mentally the best she has ever been, and wiser in her years, serving as an oracle to those who are just beginning the journey.

I want her to enjoy her life with her partner, who's doing the same thing. So when they're eighty-five or ninety-five, and they want to be intimate, they want to hang out, they can do all the things they want to do because their physiological and chemistry are youthful, and (this is the best part) they also have the benefit of having eight decades of wisdom.

It is notable to recall that when the eleventh-century knights embarked on their Crusades, the elders led the quest. Younger whippersnappers came along to prove themselves. The leaders were the purest and most capable and perhaps the men with the most testosterone.

I do not need to tell you that unless you intervene in your most-certainly-to-arise hormone deficiency, both women and men will have diminished physical functions and greater vulnerability to injury and illness in aging if you sleep through the quest for the Holy Grail. That includes testosterone, we must remind everyone, vital to a woman's health.

It may mean a foray into the undesigned-but-evolved-wrongly medical system we live with, but you should know your testosterone level.

You know what? Bioidentical hormone replacement therapy, which is best started early in life, mitigates every adverse event I have mentioned. Keeping youthful chemistry throughout your life will impact every single one of these. Your hormones represent the indispensable foundation of your health.

HORMONES OF PUBERTY AND ADOLESCENCE

Typically, the onset of puberty is the first major challenge young girls face. Sometimes they pace through their shifting hormones and the changes to their skin, hair, and breasts, but many become obsessed with the internal and external changes happening without much warning.

Hey, having your period every month, experiencing your body's changes with your breasts and hair and all those things—there's psychological development in that. These moments should be nurtured, and young girls should feel encouraged about this great time in life. This is not a curse.

"Adolescence" describes the phase of life between childhood and adulthood, and its definition has been debated for decades. Adolescence encompasses biological growth and major social role transitions, which have changed in the past century.

The Lancet published a journal article in 2018 entitled "The Age of Adolescence," suggesting that "rather than age 10–19 years, a definition of 10–24 years corresponds more closely to adolescent growth and popular understandings of this life phase and would facilitate extended investments across a broader range of settings."[128]

How Children Became "Teenagers"

In the nineteenth century, the American world consisted of children and adults. *US History* published a fascinating internet article entitled "The Invention of the Teenager," which notes that most Americans tried their best to allow their children to enjoy their youth. At the same time, they were slowly preparing for the trials and tribulations of adulthood. Although child labor practices still existed in the nineteenth century, more and more states were passing restrictions against such exploitation.

The whole world of children changed. A new category of maturity arose: the teenager.

"The average number of years spent in school for young Americans was also on the rise. Parents were waiting longer to goad their youngsters into marriage rather than pairing them off at the tender age of sixteen or seventeen. In short, it soon became apparent that a new stage of life—the *teenage* phase—was becoming a reality in America," *US History* recalls.[129]

American adolescents were displaying traits unknown among children and adults. Although the word "teenager" did not come into use until decades later, the teenage mindset dawned in the 1920s, when the word adolescent came into vogue. Then came cars, and the deal was sealed.

As teenagers emerge from childhood, hormones start the reproductive cycle and reveal secondary sexual characteristics such as axillary hair (armpits), pubic hair, and breast development, which we call *thelarche*. Then when the girl starts her period, we call that phase the *menarche*. So this accumulation of changes heralds this beautiful, detailed system kicking in, which will last for about thirty-five years.

Estrogen has become the most crucial hormone now. But we must remember that estrogen comes from testosterone. Without the production of testosterone, there is no estrogen.

Adolescence reminds me of Hans Christian Anderson's 1833 beloved fairy tale "The Ugly Duckling."

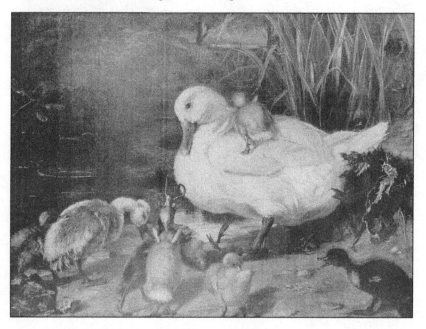

The Ugly Duckling, by Henrietta Ward

I never dreamed of such happiness as this,
while I was an ugly duckling.

—HANS CHRISTIAN ANDERSEN, "THE UGLY DUCKLING"

Girls may be awkward, feel clumsy, or view themselves as unpretty. So did Hans Christian Anderson's character the ugly duckling, whom the ducks in his family did not accept because he was different. But later, when he catches sight of his reflection in the water, he realizes he is not an ugly duckling anymore but a beautiful, elegant swan. Having discovered his beauty and found his family, this majestic swan takes flight with the flock of swans, happy at last.[130]

But like our hero, the ugly duckling's difficult journey to becoming a swan, *becoming* a woman can be challenging physically and emotionally. Hormone changes occur over a two-to three-year span in this cute little girl. This is the time when they're probably going to be their unhappiest. They may think their nose is too big, or their breasts are this or that. But it's like the swan. The ugly duckling is not a duck; it's a swan. They are caught up in a change, a new stage of growth. And I think it's a great stage to embrace change, a skill that will be very useful in the years ahead.

Cultural acknowledgment of the arrival of a girl's first period varies immensely across the globe. Stigmas and taboos still exist around the planet.

One of the most meaningful traditions is in Fiji, where communities lay out a special mat for girls during their first period and teach girls about the importance of this milestone. On the fourth day of their period, the occasion called "tundra," the girls' families prepare a feast to celebrate their daughters' entry into womanhood.[131]

The Native American tribes in North America pay tribute to girls reaching puberty with a celebration called the Sunrise Ceremony. The ceremony involves different rituals where girls from the tribe receive and offer gifts. The girls wear symbolic outfits and celebrate with a feast. Our native cultures consider the shift from childhood to adulthood as a critical moment in their children's lives, and they observe several coming-of-age rites to assert their traditional and community values.[132]

We should also prepare feasts of celebration. All of a sudden, young girls become young women. I recall a 2022 TV series title that says it all, and very likely instantly, brings back deep-seated memories in many women: *The Summer I Turned Pretty*. Adolescent girls experience a curving of the hips and forming of the mammary. Their limbs lengthen until estrogen stops the formation of the epiphyseal plate within the bone and stops the growth. That's why boys' limbs grow longer; they grow taller later in adolescence when their testosterone makes enough estrogen to close that plate.

The side effects of these new sexual characteristics—the acne, the hair, the breasts, and the changing of their cycles—are not clinical subjects for treatment. But I want that embraced as a wonderful time of life. They're leaving this beautiful childhood, and now they're entering this area of becoming beautiful women with all the strength they need.

Acne is not fun, but it is not a hormonal issue. I see young girls with very low testosterone who have bad acne. It's a gut issue. Skin, gut, and brain go together in the immune system. Those three systems are tied together. It's a triad. A healthy diet and a healthy gut are the best remedies.

Estrogen, testosterone, and progesterone have key roles in our sex differentiation from the womb and throughout life. Our hormones guide every event from that miraculous moment of inception: egg production, fertility, sexual characteristics, defense of the fetus, maturing into a child, then an adolescent, then an adult. This is by design and not by accident, and hormones stay in the center of the rest of life. It stretches our capacity to wonder to contemplate the continuous metamorphosis of the female human body.

The Mayo Clinic reminds us of the fact that during our life journey, females are more than twice as likely as males to suffer from anxiety and depression.[133] Why? Testosterone yields protective benefits against both. Decreased levels of testosterone create a significantly higher presence of anxiety and depression. Many studies show that hormone replacement therapy dramatically improves mood, alleviates stress, and mitigates symptoms of depression. Additionally, as I have mentioned, BHRT may protect against heart attacks, disease, dementia, and osteoporosis and help heal post-traumatic stress disorder (PTSD) and traumatic brain injury (TBI).[134]

HORMONES AFFECTING FERTILITY

Childbearing age, culturally in America, can begin as early as age eleven or twelve. That's the physical part. The mental part, not so much.

Precocious Puberty

Thelarche is a medical term referring to the appearance of breast development in girls, usually occurring after age eight, accompanied by other signs of puberty, including a growth spurt. In America, we see precocious puberty earlier and earlier due to, I believe, our endocrine disruptors. We all are being exposed to fake estrogens in the environment. Our bodies cannot distinguish the good ones from the bad ones, so these characteristics, like early breast formation, and early cycles, begin because of our very bad, processed food and our high grain and sugar consumption. This leads to increased production of these fake estrogens that trick the body into kicking in some secondary characteristics.

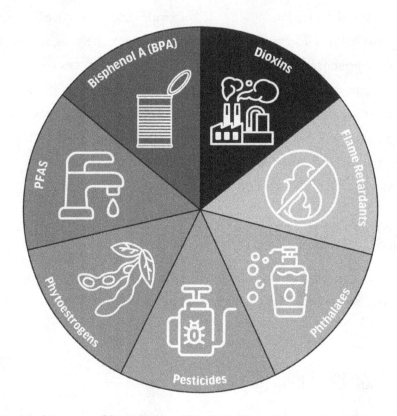

National Institute of Environmental Health Sciences, "Endocrine Disruptors,
https://www.niehs.nih.gov/health/topics/agents/endocrine/index.cfm, accessed August 11, 2023.
National Institute of Environmental Health Sciences Endocrine Disruptors

Our ugly duckling is not yet a swan when stepping into child-bearing age. She has lived with awkwardness and poor self-image, and suddenly, she discovers that she has become attractive. Hormonally, things are happening.

Your FSH (follicle-stimulating hormone) comes from the anterior pituitary gland, which stimulates the ovary to make testosterone, which turns into estrogen, vital to a healthy life.

Unlike men, who continue to produce sperm throughout their lives, a woman is born with all the egg-containing follicles in her ovaries that she will ever have. At birth, there are about one million follicles. That number will have dropped to around three hundred thousand as puberty arrives.

Several hundred will be ovulated during the reproductive years. As the estrogen level gets high enough, the estradiol stimulates the anterior pituitary to release LH (luteinizing hormone) to make progesterone. Luteinizing hormone is produced by the pituitary gland and is one of the main hormones that control the reproductive system.

The Society for Endocrinology describes this amazing process:

> In women, luteinizing hormone carries out different roles in the two halves of the menstrual cycle. In weeks one to two of the cycle, luteinizing hormone is required to stimulate the ovarian follicles in the ovary to produce the female sex hormone estradiol. Around day 14 of the cycle, a surge in luteinizing hormone levels causes the ovarian follicle to rupture and release a mature oocyte (egg) from the ovary, a process called ovulation. For the remainder of the cycle (weeks three to four), the remnants of the ovarian follicle form a corpus luteum. The luteinizing hormone stimulates the corpus luteum to produce progesterone, which is required to support the early stages of pregnancy if fertilization occurs.[135]

What does that mean? Pro-gestation. Prolife. That's what progesterone means: prolife. Hold that baby in the womb. That's its job. That's what's happening now in the second part of the month, and if you're pregnant, the placenta will continue to make progesterone throughout the pregnancy. Progesterone goes higher. If you're not pregnant, it goes down, and you start the cycle again.

The American Society for Reproductive Medicine observes that a woman's best reproductive years are in her twenties. Fertility gradually declines in the thirties, especially after age thirty-five. Each month that she tries, a healthy, fertile thirty-year-old woman has a 20 percent chance of getting pregnant.[136] That means that for every one hundred fertile thirty-year-old women trying to get pregnant in one cycle, twenty will be successful, and the other eighty will have to try again. By age forty, a woman's chance is less than 5 percent per cycle, so fewer than five out of every one hundred women are expected to be successful each month.

So it begins in adolescence, this extraordinary period of protecting life. Usually, hormones are at the optimal range. The key is, if your periods are regular, you're in an optimal range. It's the outside influences that throw the cycles off, such as emotional stress, and high sugar intake. So if a woman's cycle is not regular, that is a sign that she's not hormonally balanced.

Plenty of Estrogens

In their fertility range, women usually have plenty of estrogen, maybe too much, and progesterone. Just like men, their problem is testosterone. Women need testosterone as well. The brain tells the testicle or ovary, whichever the case may be, to make testosterone first, which then converts to estrogen. So when caring for younger women with brain fog, tiredness, or decreased libido, I always look at their testosterone and thyroid levels.

Follicle-Stimulating Hormone (FSH)

During their reproductive years, women have regular monthly menstrual periods because they ovulate regularly each month. Eggs mature inside fluid-filled spheres called "follicles." At the beginning of each menstrual cycle, when a woman is having her period, a hormone produced in the pituitary gland, which is in the brain, stimulates a group of follicles to grow more rapidly on both ovaries.

The pituitary hormone that stimulates the ovaries is called follicle-stimulating hormone (FSH). Typically, only one of those follicles will reach maturity and release an egg (ovulate); the remainder gradually will stop growing and degenerate. Pregnancy results if the egg becomes fertilized and implants in the lining of the uterus (endometrium).

If pregnancy does not occur, the endometrium is shed as the menstrual flow and the cycle begins again. In their early teens, girls often have irregular ovulation resulting in irregular menstrual cycles, but by age sixteen, they should have established regular ovulation resulting in regular periods. A woman's cycles will remain regular, twenty-six to thirty-five days, until her late thirties to early forties, when she may notice that her cycles become shorter. As time passes, she will begin to skip ovulation resulting in missed periods. Ultimately, periods become increasingly infrequent until they cease completely.[137]

The best hormonal status you can have can be illustrated by a twenty-three-year-old woman with regular cycles who eats, exercises, and sleeps well. That's optimal. We're always looking to get to that. And it's not because we want to be young, and we don't want to age. No, no, no. We love aging. We love the matchless wisdom that comes with age—we just don't want the diseases that come with it. That's why we monitor hormones regularly even at a seemingly optimal age. I tell my patients never to accept that we all are destined to have chronic diseases. The evidence is in. We're not.

Testosterone

Women aged twenty to forty lose half of their testosterone, affecting reproduction, mood, motivation, brain health, breast health, bone density, muscle mass, and vascular health. Lifestyle factors can also contribute to low T, such as lack of exercise, statin drugs, stress, and nutrient deficiencies. This sets up low sexual desire and arousal, fatigue, bone loss, muscle weakness, weight gain, and decreased lean body mass.[138]

Most women feel great in their luteal phase, the second half of the menstrual cycle. Still, there can be mood changes, changes in sexual desire, bloating, breast swelling, pain or tenderness, headache, weight fluctuations, food cravings, or trouble sleeping. None of these should indicate the use of mental health medications.

IT'S ALL IN YOUR HEAD

There can be problems all along this journey. One of my patients is a beautiful twenty-five-year-old woman, who loves her husband, has no libido, and has anxiety and menstrual discomfort. Her gynecologist has told her, "It's just part of being a woman. It's all in your head."

That drives me nuts. *No, no, no.* There's no way. Something is going on here in this woman's body at the biochemical level, and this is not unusual. And if it is in their head, it's because that's where their brain is, not because it's make-believe out of thin air. *Here's another pill. Here's your fluoxetine.*

The first thing we need to check, after a history and physical, and a look at her diet and the medications she is taking, are the hormone levels. These symptoms can be remedied but not by drugs that can mess you up even more.

You're a swan, not an ugly duckling.

Hormones in Childbirth

Dramatic decreases in several hormones accompany pregnancy and childbirth, such as estradiol, progesterone, and cortisol. Reproductive hormones and stress hormones rise dramatically during pregnancy and then drop suddenly upon delivery.

Odds are a family's first baby can be the most challenging. It's the fear of the unknown. The first delivery is usually the most complicated.

For subsequent children, much of the anxiousness is decreased. Once you have accomplished the process once, it may seem easier. Many times, the second, third, and fourth babies are easier for the mom. The newborn arrives to a much more relaxed vibe. *Been there, done that.*

The correct balance of hormones is essential for a successful pregnancy. Hormones act as the body's chemical messengers sending information and feeding back responses between different tissues and organs. Hormones travel around the body, usually in the blood, and attach to proteins on the cells called receptors, much like a key fits a lock or a hand fits a glove.

The Society for Endocrinology describes that "in response to this, the target tissue or organ functions in a way that ensures pregnancy is maintained. Initially, the ovaries, and then later, the placenta, are the main producers of pregnancy-related hormones that are essential in creating and maintaining the correct conditions required for a successful pregnancy."[139]

The thyroid hormones also completely change as well during that postpartum state. Mom can get what's called postpartum thyrotoxicosis. She can have a very, very high thyroid or very, very low thyroid.

The cause of postpartum blues, I believe, is because of a rapid loss of hormones. That's the issue. I've placed bioidentical pellets and given the needed testosterone a touch of estrogen, so it does not affect the milk supply. Within a couple of days, the postpartum blues and depression end.

The blues may be predicted by watching for lower levels of the hormone allopregnanolone in the second trimester of pregnancy, a subject under clinical study associated with an increased chance of developing postpartum depression (PPD) in women already known to be at risk for the disorder.[140]

Postpartum depression affects early bonding between the mother and child. This should be treated because the implications for the mother and baby can be severe. While baby blues syndrome does not require treatment, postpartum depression is a serious, potentially life-threatening condition that does require a doctor's attention. The mainstream treatment for PPD generally includes prescribing antidepressants.[141]

Yet only 15 percent of women with postpartum depression are estimated to ever receive professional treatment, according to the US Centers for Disease Control and Prevention. Many physicians don't screen for it, and there seems to be a stigma for mothers. A mother who asks for help may be seen as incapable of handling her situation as a mother, or friends or family may criticize her for taking medication during or shortly after pregnancy. Postpartum women may prefer natural alternatives, especially those who breastfeed their infants.[142]

In my thirty years as an OB/GYN, I view the cause of PPD as a drop in maternal hormones (especially progesterone) after labor and delivery. Therefore, supplementing with bioidentical progesterone to help replace that rapid loss, I have found to vastly improve and even cure PPD symptoms in many women.

We also keep a close eye on your thyroid, iodine production, vitamin D, and hormone replacement postpartum. (There's more on this in chapters 7 and 8.)

Many women are waiting to start their families for many reasons. Marriages occur later in life than in the past. Many women place high priorities on their careers. There are economic concerns with the costs of raising a child. And even though we have seen a significant trend of women taking better care of themselves in recent years, there is still a natural age-related decline in fertility, directly related to the number of eggs that remain in her ovaries. This decline may take place much sooner than most women expect. Menopause is defined as the absence of menstrual periods for one year when no other cause can be identified. (It is often accompanied by symptoms such as hot flashes and night sweats.)

> "I have my hormones balanced. Most doctors are giving women synthetic hormones, which just eliminate the symptoms, but it's doing nothing to actually replace the hormones you have lost. Without our hormones, we die."[143]
>
> —SUZANNE SOMERS

Hormones in Midlife

So we go from the strain of childbearing and parenting into the thirties and forties, and women are obsessed over losing baby weight after having their children. Baby weight is hormonal because, again, when you have a high estrogen level (E1) stored in fat, that propagates a catch-22 of increasing fat.

Changes in the bacteria in your gut, and estrogen metabolites, cause a reaction of keeping more fat.

At this time, thyroids usually get out of whack, as does testosterone. Picture this: you have matured into this phase, now a forty-five-year-old woman, also dealing with a fourteen-year-old hormonal boy or girl. It's all over again—the same cycle.

Today, age-related infertility is becoming more common because, for various reasons, many women wait until their thirties to begin their families. Even though some women today are healthier and taking better care of themselves than ever before, improved health in later life does not offset the natural age-related decline in fertility. It is essential to understand that fertility declines as a woman ages due to the average age-related decrease in the number of eggs that remain in her ovaries. This decline may take place much sooner than most women expect.

Women do not remain fertile until menopause. The average age for menopause is fifty-one, but most women cannot have a successful pregnancy until sometime in their midforties at the latest. These percentages are true for natural conception as well as conception using fertility treatment, including in vitro fertilization (IVF). Although stories in the news media may lead women and their partners to believe that they can use fertility treatments such as IVF to get pregnant, a woman's age affects the success rates of infertility treatments. The age-related loss of female fertility happens because the quality and the number of eggs gradually decline. That has to do with, again, testosterone.

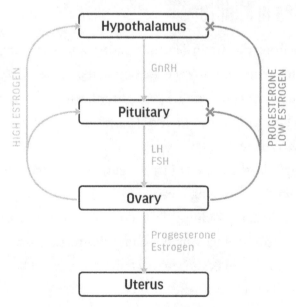

HORMONES AND VISIBLE CONFIDENCE

There's confidence in womanhood. There's no doubt about it. Our natural hormones blur our functions. It does not mean a man can't cook. It does not imply that a woman can't own a company. It does not represent any of that. It just means that to be your potential, your best, you learn to exude confidence.

People instantly recognize a strong woman, a strong mom, a confident woman, when she walks into the room. She doesn't have to say a thing. Watch a female congresswoman enter a room. Watch people react to a female four-star general. Look closely at a strong mother, an assertive teacher, a female marine, a female firefighter, or a female police officer. It's not the job. Their strength comes from within. They do not have to do or say a thing. There are hormonal and decision-making differences between men and women, but the unique strength of feminine strength cannot be denied.

In every case, a woman with an aura of strength effortlessly exudes that vibe because she has optimal hormone levels.

I recently performed a pellet placement for a thirty-five-year-old female executive who, months before, was skeptical. At the time, she told me, "I'm here, Greg, because I was a skeptic, but after my husband's placement, I saw a big difference." So she decided to have bioidentical hormone replacement. She became a believer.

After her third placement visit, she said, "Everyone should have this. This is a breakthrough in every way."

Very recently, a forty-two-year-old lady, whom I had worked with for three years, came in with irregular bleeding.

"It cannot be from pellet placement," I told her, "because you're not getting estrogen right now. I'm just giving you testosterone."

She had first come to us following fourteen years of depression and traumatic births, and all her doctors wanted to give her was antidepressants. She found us and has been off antidepressants ever since. After her first pellet placement, she became a new person. Her libido's back, her life's back, and she's in great shape.

"I feel phenomenal," she reiterated every time she came in.

So why the bleeding? I walked her through the structure. About 85 percent of irregular bleeding is hormonal. If it's not hormonal, 15 percent is structural, usually a tiny polyp or fibroid.

She understood all that and returned to her doctor, telling him it was a polyp. The doctor said again, "It's the hormones, the pellets."

She replied, "No, it isn't."

Her physician gave her an alternative. "You have to choose. Please stay on the pellets or do my plan. Go back on the happy pills."

And she replied, "And have no libido, no life, because I have a tiny structural defect?"

This gal knew how to defend her *medical freedom*.

We spent some time talking, and she said, "I cannot believe them. I've been in their hands for fourteen years, and they did nothing for me. The last three years have been the best years of my life, and all because I got this small little polyp; all I needed was a small biopsy, and my doctor insists that I discontinue the hormone therapy."

That's often the mantra: *It's all in your head. Here's a sertraline HCl, here's a fluoxetine, here's your mood swing.* I was like that doctor years ago. I prescribed vitamin D, fish oil, and probiotics, and occasionally I offered these remedies. No longer. We have better answers now. We use bioidentical hormones, and we still love probiotics, vitamin D, and fish oil as well.

She had very, very bad postpartum depression, too, before she came to us. I wish I had known her then. I could have taken care of that with pellets because these problems are not make-believe. They are real issues with real root causes. These pills are putting band-aids on the symptoms, not thoughtfully looking for the root cause. The root cause is the need for hormonal restoration, in midlife, in the perimenopausal state, in the postpartum state, in a menopausal state, in depression, anxiety, look there. There's a new answer to most of this.

We now know that estrogen, testosterone, and progesterone make the nerves neuroplastic, allow the synapsis to talk, and make everything healthier in the brain.

So this roller coaster, these incredible women, these beautiful gifts from God, are on is almost continuous. And now they're reaching the end of their childbearing age, and they've had their family, and what's the first symptom that that's all over?

Here come hot flashes and mood changes. People call them *normal*.

Researchers have begun to pay more attention to cardiovascular risk factors unique to women, such as early menopause (before age forty) and certain pregnancy complications. Recently they turned their attention to this common menopausal symptom that affects up to 85 percent of women.[144]

Study results were presented in September 2019 to the North American Menopause Society from the Study of Women's Health Across the Nation (SWAN). Researchers found that women who experience frequent or persistent hot flashes may be likelier than women who don't to experience a heart attack, stroke, or other serious cardiovascular problems. (Researchers defined "frequent" hot flashes as having them six or more days in the previous two-week period. Women with "persistent" hot flashes reported those frequent hot flashes at 25 percent or more of study visits.[145])

Once you start having perimenopausal symptoms, I'm not saying it's too late, but you need to have an awakening that damage may be occurring. Medicine should not disregard these symptoms just because it does not involve fertility.

SCIENTISTS AND RESEARCHERS ARE ASSEMBLING CONVINCING EVIDENCE OBSERVING SEX HORMONES AS A PROTECTION AGAINST DEMENTIA, PARKINSON'S, AND ALZHEIMER'S

Perimenopause and Menopause Seen
as Critical Tipping Points

Some of the most compelling research in the life-changing hormone therapy comes from a 2018 academic endocrinology book entitled Sex *Hormones in Neurodegenerative Processes and Diseases*, edited by Gorazd Drevenšek, MSc, PhD.

Gorazd Drevenšek holds an MSc degree in Pharmacology and a PhD degree in medical sciences, both from the University of Ljubljana, Faculty of Medicine. He started his research in cardiovascular pharmacology, modeling ischemic and reperfusion injuries and atherosclerotic processes. His focus is on the pharmacological and toxicological evaluation of natural compounds as potential therapeutic agents with cardio–and neuro-protectant potential.

Dr. Drevenšek assembled recent evidence from throughout the medical world, focused on neurodegenerative diseases, one of the main global burdens and one of the public health priorities everywhere. And it's getting worse because the population is aging.

The fourteen chapters sum up the past and current knowledge on sex hormones, representing original new insights into their role in brain functioning, mental disorders, and neurodegenerative diseases. The book is written for a broad range of audiences, from biomedical students to highly profiled medical specialists and biomedical researchers, helping them to expand their knowledge on sex hormones in neurodegenerative processes and opening new questions for further investigation.[146]

One of the main differences between the male and female population "appears due to sex hormone alterations that affect the initiation of neurodegenerative processes," he summarizes.[147]

"The potential therapeutic role in neurodegenerative processes has been largely neglected in comparison to other therapeutic research," Dr. Drevenšek adds.[148]

- "Non-genomic action of sex hormones, their protective role in their modulatory effects on neural tissues are becoming more important with epidemiological data on the sex-related differences. Also, sex hormones acting as neuroactive steroids show pleiotropic effects that enable neuroprotection, neuroplasticity, neuron survival, and regeneration and reduce excitotoxicity.[149]

In other words, research continues to be quite promising as regards the ability of sex hormones to halt or delay dementia, Alzheimer's, and other disorders of the brain.

- "Cognitive decline, age-related neurological disorders and dementia and others may, in part at least, be attributed to decreased secretion of DHEA that acts probably through diminished glutamate-induced excitotoxicity."[150]

In other words, science continues to link Alzheimer's with hormone depletion. The book offers new insights into the "potential for hormone replacement therapy during perimenopause to be a potential protectant against Alzheimer's disease."[151]

- There has been shown to be a higher incidence of Parkinson's disease present in postmenopausal compared to premenopausal women of similar age, suggesting that estrogens do possess neuroprotective effects.[152]

- This collection of the latest science explores perimenopause as a "critical period" in neuro-aging, when the neurodegenerative processes may initiate.[153]

- Estrogens delay the onset of frontotemporal dementia (FTLD) in premenopausal women compared to age-equivalent men and may provide neuroprotection in the early postmenopausal period.[154]

Note: Each chapter in this open-access, peer-reviewed landmark book can be downloaded and enjoyed at no cost by visiting the IntechOpen website listed in the footnote.

So why don't we keep her bones strong like a twenty-five-year-old? Why don't we keep her brain as quick as a twenty-five-year-old? Yes, her baby-making years are gone. She is through that phase. Let's keep her heart healthy. If you picture life on a scale, one end is when she's born. On the other end, she goes to heaven. In the middle is menopause. Miles to go before we sleep. Stop saying her pain is normal. A BHRT program will mitigate all the hot flashes and mood swings. Just replace the missing estrogen.

Which hormone dominates before menopause in the estrogen family? It's estradiol. Which one dominates in the menopausal state?

Estrone (E1), estradiol (E2), and estriol (E3) are three endogenously produced estrogens. Estradiol (E2) is produced by the dominant ovarian follicle during the monthly menstrual cycle and is the most potent natural estrogen. Estrone (E1) is the dominant form of estrogen during menopause. It is produced in small quantities by the ovary and the adrenal glands and is principally derived by the peripheral conversion of androstenedione in adipose tissue.[155]

Where are the heart attacks on the menopausal side? Where is breast cancer on the menopausal side? Where's stroke, dementia, and osteoporosis? Why? Up until this point, your hormones have protected you. The dominant one, testosterone, which makes cells healthy, is not there. And the one that is there is a five to one alpha growth that increases disease. Same thing with the male's prostate. So the answer is, I see no benefit of having low "hormones for your age."

In medicine, sex hormones have a special status. They are the only hormones that luminaries quantify based on your age.

We do not say, "That's a healthy insulin for a diabetic or a healthy insulin for your age."

Age is irrelevant to blood sugar. Blood sugar over 95 is terrible, period. And today's insulin has left the barnyard behind. It's all bioidentical now. To get the exact structure, we make it from bacteria, e. coli. All hormone replacement should be done with bioidentical hormones.

So there's an *uh-oh moment* when women notice their fine lines and wrinkles signaling that they're aging. It comes around about this time for many folks.

I have some peptides for that. (Please see more on peptides in chapter 8.) When your estrogen and your progesterone, a testosterone, are higher, you make better collagen, and you don't get wrinkles. There's a property of peptide that helps that collagen to strengthen. It's almost like having surgery without having surgery.

A question remains. Moods, depression, vaginal dryness, bladder infections, loss of bone, increased heart attack risk, and osteoporosis arrive. So are we manipulating nature by keeping the hormone levels optimal?

I can see people arguing that we are messing with nature. *It's naturally getting old.* I got that. But I think it's part of our brain being used, what God gave us. We cannot extend the reproductive age, even if there are ways to keep the cells healthy. But we can extend the reproductive hormonal benefits. That's aging gracefully. It's not trying to recapture youthful body chemistry to have babies. It's recapturing the ability to take advantage of the wisdom of age with a healthy brain, body, and outlook.

Centers for Disease Control

LEADING CAUSES OF DEATH:
Females of All Races, Ages, and Origins

Heart disease 21.8%

Cancer 20.7%

Respiratory diseases 6.2%

Stroke 6.2%

Alzheimer's disease 6.1%

Unintentional injuries 4.4%

Diabetes 2.7%

Influenza and pneumonia 2.1%[156]

Heart disease and cancer rank at the top of the causes of death in women.

Both genetics and lifestyle significantly influence the risk of cancer. While individuals can modify their lifestyle, culture and environment can hinder some progress in reducing lifestyle-related cancer risks.

According to an article published by the Roswell Park Cancer Institute, these factors may explain why American women are up to five times more likely to be diagnosed with breast cancer.

"In general, one out of eight women in the US will be diagnosed with breast cancer in their lifetime," said Kazuki Takabe, MD, clinical chief of Breast Surgery at Roswell Park Cancer Institute. "In Japan, that is one out of every thirty-eight, but it was even less a decade ago."[157]

American women generally consume more saturated fats and drink more alcohol compared with Japanese women, according to the authors. Japanese women tend to eat diets high in soy, walk more, and have children later.

These lifestyle factors have been known to cause a significant gap in breast cancer rates between the two countries; however, the rate of breast cancer has been increasing in Japan. This change has been speculated to be the result of Western influence.

The fact is that three or four decades ago, "there was less breast cancer in Japan, so there must be some environmental changes that are causing this," Dr. Takabe said. "It's been said that the Western lifestyle and diet contribute to this high incidence rate. In Japan, as the younger generations are adopting the American culture, diet, and habits, the breast cancer rate is increasing."[158]

Pharmacy Times writer Laurie Torch asked, "What do they do differently?"[159]

They take vitamin B at a higher rate and have two hundred times higher levels of iodine.[160]

"When America ate that much iodine fifty years ago, our breast cancer rate was one in twenty. There are many benefits to protecting glandular cells. It's called the sodium iodine system. It makes glandular cells healthier." (More on iodine and Vitamin B in chapters 7 and 8.)

I see multiple reasons for this. We've had all these years of genetics proving that it may not be cancer; it might be just the environment causing the cells to go out of order. The biggest culprit is sugar. How do we make this beautiful Ferrari, our body, cope in a hostile environment? Let's get the immune system, the muscle system, the energy system, the heart system, and the neuro system as aggressive as possible for this hostile environment. Then we're surviving. Now we're thriving, regardless of age.

DANGERS OF SYNTHETIC HORMONES ARE NOW CLEAR

Some time has passed since the influential 2002 WHI study, but new research from the same organization continues to shed important light on the risks of synthetic hormones. The organization's February 2010 study showed that hormone therapy using a combination of synthetic progestin with estrogen confirmed short-term heart disease risks for postmenopausal women.

Synthetic hormones are not natural. Does it make sense to introduce a chemical long-term that is entirely unfamiliar to your genetic makeup? Premarin is obviously synthetic, derived from pregnant horse urine. Provera is another synthetic chemical made from medroxyprogesterone acetate, which is a chemical derivative of progesterone. A high percentage of women who start taking these drugs discover the side effects are so uncomfortable that they discontinue use.

In 2019, The *British Medical Journal* published a commentary about hormone replacement therapy and breast cancer risk and commented on HRT and breast cancer risk, progesterone vs. progestins.

"Evidence suggests that there are important differences in breast cancer risks with different progestogens used in combined (oestrogen

+ progestogen) hormone replacement therapy (HRT) regimens; micronized natural/bioidentical progesterone appears to be a far safer choice than synthetic progestins."[161]

A large French study which assessed and compared the association between different HRTs and breast cancer risk, followed 80,377 women for an average of 8.1 postmenopausal years, and found that compared with HRT never-use, there was no increased risk of breast cancer for oestrogen-progesterone (relative risk 1.00), whereas those using oestrogen plus progestins had a relative risk of 1.16-1.69 (depending on the progestin used).[162]

Bioidentical, natural hormones are a "far safer choice."

Another French study also found that breast cancer risk differed by type of progestogen among current users of estrogen-progestogen therapies. No increased risk was apparent among users of estrogen + micronized natural progesterone for any duration (odds ratio 0.80), whereas among users of combined HRT containing a synthetic progestin, the odds ratio was 1.57–3.35 (depending on the progestin used).[163]

A meta-analysis of studies of postmenopausal women using progesterone versus synthetic progestins in combination with estrogen found that progesterone-estrogen was associated with a lower risk of breast cancer compared with synthetic progestins (relative risk 0.67).

MENTAL HEALTH

What's the most challenging phase in a woman's life? What is the role of our hormones in keeping females well-balanced through all this change?

It's normal to be on antidepressants. According to *NBC News*, one in six Americans takes some kind of psychiatric drug.[164]

It's normal to be tired. *Ah, don't worry. It's just in your head.* This is an organic function. The brain operates better when it's hormonally optimized. Period. Mental health challenges affect women of all ages.

The top two reasons why people come to us—whether they are an eighteen-year-old man, twenty-five-year-old woman, sixty-year-old guy, or seventy-five-year-old woman—have stayed steady for over ten years: tired of being tired and brain fog. Number three is anxiety and depression. Number four is loss of energy and motivation. Number five is libido.

Can you be low on hormones when you're eighteen or twenty-five? Yeah, you can. We're getting bombarded by the environment. This new generation is starting at a lower point. So if these hormones help mental capabilities and if they're a lower value and the brain's not optimal, you'll have these symptoms earlier.

I used to think these things would rise later in life. Not anymore. It's directly related to life stresses. So I think the hormone panel is the first thing we must evaluate at every age. Compare that to a previous panel, if available, to see what level they experienced, perhaps not as influenced by these neuroendocrine disruptors.

We know starting to replace your hormones when transitioning in that stage is far superior because you'll never have symptoms. My wife has no idea what a hot flash is. Never, never. She has no idea what vaginal dryness is. She has no idea of any perimenopausal or menopausal symptoms. And by her age, she had been going through this for the last fifteen years.

Hormone changes can happen much earlier these days, up to a decade or more before the symptoms of no periods.

My message here is to not wait for something to go wrong. Do you want the body, brain, immune system, and cardiovascular system of a twenty-five-year-old? Or do you want those of an eighty-year-old?

PERIMENOPAUSE

Perimenopause is the transitional time around menopause. Menopause is when a woman's periods stop. It's marked by changes in the menstrual cycle and other physical and emotional symptoms. Johns Hopkins Medicine notes that this time can last two to ten years.

PERIMENOPAUSE

Johns Hopkins Medicine

During this time, your body:

- Releases eggs less regularly
- Produces less estrogen and other hormones
- Becomes less fertile
- Has shorter and more irregular menstrual cycles

Perimenopause is a natural process caused as your ovaries gradually stop working. Ovulation may become erratic and then stop. The menstrual cycle lengthens, and flow may become irregular before your final period.[165]

The changing levels of hormones in the body cause symptoms. When estrogen is higher, you may have symptoms as you might have with PMS. When estrogen is low, you may have hot flashes or night sweats. These hormone changes may be mixed with normal cycles.

In perimenopause, women start losing progesterone first, then estrogen second. We can see those values in blood tests. Then in menopause, they've lost everything. By strict definition, menopause arrives after one year of no periods. We know that 5 percent of bone loss can start during the perimenopausal range. Other troubling issues arise, such as hot flashes, decreased coronary vessels' elasticity, and brain communication with the body.

When symptoms happen, you need to catch them. When you cease making estradiol, the brain produces more FSH to try to turn on the ovaries' production of estrogen. It can't, but it tries to. And the higher the FSH is, the more the symptoms. Also, that can happen even when you have periods; you're just not making enough estrogen.

WHAT ARE THE SYMPTOMS OF PERIMENOPAUSE?
No two women will experience perimenopause in the same way.

These are the most common symptoms:

- Mood changes
- Changes in sexual desire
- Trouble concentrating
- Headaches
- Night sweats
- Hot flashes
- Vaginal dryness
- Trouble with sleep
- Joint and muscle aches
- Heavy sweating
- Having to pee often
- PMS-like symptoms[166]

MENOPAUSE

Julia Prague of *Nature* recently looked at the book *The Slow Moon Climbs: The Science, History, and Meaning of Menopause*, by Susan P. Mattern, who observed that in the 1820s, the French physician Charles-Pierre-Louis de Gardanne coined the term menopause.

"By 1899, the US pharmaceuticals company Merck was selling Ovariin, a treatment derived from dried and pulverized bovine ovaries. Over a century of trials and treatments, the medical understanding of menopause has advanced significantly (although not nearly enough), even as cultural attitudes to it have shifted," Mattern observed.[167]

In her book *The Slow Moon Climbs*, historian Susan Mattern seeks to change the perception of menopause, stressing the natural-selective advantage of living well beyond the reproductive years.

Me too.

The average age for menopause is fifty-one, but the age range most often referred to is between forty-five and fifty-five. During this time, as in perimenopause, women start losing progesterone first and then estrogen. We can see those values based on blood tests. And then, once entirely in menopause, they've lost everything.

Why do women begin having the same health crises as men as soon as the hormones go away? They've lost their protective hormones. What about osteoporosis? Breast cancer? Strokes? Up until menopause, the protective properties of hormones have protected women.

Heart disease in women is a deep concern around the world. The worldwide INTERHEART Study, a large cohort study of more than fifty-two thousand individuals with myocardial infarction, have revealed that women have their first presentation of coronary heart disease approximately ten years later than men, most commonly after menopause. Despite this delay in onset, mortality is increasing more rapidly among women than men.[168]

So before menopause, a woman's chance of dying of a heart attack is almost zero.

But now, experiencing menopause, with hormones taken out of the picture, the chances of a woman having a heart attack are the same as a man. The American Heart Association notes that males are more prone to heart attacks than females who have not reached menopause. However, this risk is equal between males and females who have reached menopause.

Well, what did she have decades earlier? She had higher estrogen levels, testosterone levels, and progesterone levels. So it's exciting to me when we look at the data on that, we ask, what's different? They're protected. The higher estrogen and testosterone levels when they are younger shield them. When their hormone levels drop, the risk is the same as a man.

Can we push out those disease processes and eliminate some of them by restoring their youthful body chemistry? Sure. We can now.

The Endocrine Society notes that preventing bone loss is an important concern for women in the menopause journey and during postmenopausal stages.

"Menopause significantly speeds bone loss and increases the risk of osteoporosis. Research indicates that up to 20 percent of bone loss can happen during these stages and approximately one in ten women over the age of 60 are affected by osteoporosis worldwide."[169]

"One in two postmenopausal women will have osteoporosis, and most will suffer a fracture during their lifetime. Fractures (broken bones) cause pain, decreased mobility, and function. Fractures are associated with decreased quality of life and increased mortality."[170]

If you have bioidentical hormone replacement with subcutaneous pellets, you gain bone strength annually. For over twenty years, clinical studies have concluded that in fighting osteoporosis, bioidentical pellets increase bone density.

THE 2022 HORMONE THERAPY POSITION STATEMENT OF THE NORTH AMERICAN MENOPAUSE SOCIETY (NAMS)

An Advisory Panel of clinicians and research experts in the field of women's health and menopause was recruited by NAMS to review the 2017 Position Statement, evaluate new literature, assess the evidence, and reach consensus on recommendations, using the level of evidence to identify the strength of recommendations and the quality of the evidence. The Advisory Panel's recommendations were reviewed and approved by the NAMS Board of Trustees.

Hormone therapy remains the most effective treatment for vasomotor symptoms (VMS) and the genitourinary syndrome of menopause and has been shown to prevent bone loss and fracture. The risks of hormone therapy differ depending on type, dose, duration of use, route of administration, timing of initiation, and whether a progestogen is used. Treatment should be individualized using the best available evidence to maximize benefits and minimize risks, with periodic reevaluation of the benefits and risks of continuing therapy.

For women aged younger than 60 years or who are within ten years of menopause onset and have no contraindications, the benefit-risk ratio is favorable for treatment of bothersome VMS and prevention of bone loss.

> For women who initiate hormone therapy more than ten years from menopause onset or who are aged older than 60 years, the benefit-risk ratio appears less favorable because of the greater absolute risks of coronary heart disease, stroke, venous thromboembolism, and dementia. Longer durations of therapy should be for documented indications such as persistent VMS, with shared decision-making and periodic reevaluation.[171]
>
> **Source:** *The Journal of the*
> *North American Menopause Association*
> *May 2, 2022*

In that study, the risk they mention is only significant in the first six months, and after that, the risk diminishes, and the benefits are clear.

When I respond to a thirty-five-year-old mom who is forgetting words, has three kids, is always tired, and has no libido, I am reminded that 50 percent of her testosterone is gone by age forty. Symptoms of low T in women are common in their forties, fifties, and beyond. Lifestyle factors contributing to lowering testosterone levels include a lack of activity (being sedentary, statin drugs, stress, and nutrient deficiencies).

Around age fifty, women's ovaries begin producing decreasing amounts of estrogen and progesterone; the pituitary gland tries to compensate by producing more follicle-stimulating hormone (FSH).

> While menopause is normal and happens to all women, some symptoms can be irritating or dangerous. Symptoms might include the following:
>
> - Hot flashes
> - Vaginal dryness and atrophy lead to painful intercourse

- Decreased libido

- Insomnia

- Irritability/depression

- Osteoporosis can increase the likelihood of bone fractures[172]

So today, with the powerful impact of BHRT, life after age sixty can last another thirty to forty years. Within three months, the vagina returns to that of a twenty-five-year-old. The new hormones protect your heart and brain. Decades of productivity, remaining physically active and alert, helping with grandkids, and beautiful years of spiritual growth and love await.

But you must choose carefully.

HORMONES AFTER MENOPAUSE

All women breathe a sigh of relief when the menopausal symptoms conclude. But they have become more aware that chronic aches and pains will keep them from being as active as they once were or would like to be, so they make the necessary adjustments. They get screenings for heart and cancer. They alter their diet and exercise.

But it never ends. That bothers me when some experts suggest that menopause stops in three to seven years because the hot flashes stop. Menopause never really stops. Your vagina gets thinner every single day. A woman's labia majora and minora get thin. The minora goes away. The bladder can fall, you experience increased infections, and you can't have intercourse. It is not healthier to be that way.

As an OB/GYN physician, I surgically fixed those things. Even before I fixed them, I always gave my patients two months of estrogen cream to improve my surgical planes, which were very effective.

After I began to introduce my patients to testosterone for these issues, we enjoyed great results without surgery. General uterine incontinence, or prolapse, is mitigated because the anatomy gains strength. If you look under the microscope at the thinness of a vagina in menopause, you could describe it as like wet tissue paper. The thickness of a vagina of a young woman is like a wet sponge. Well, those things can happen to an eighty-year-old as well. There's no reason they cannot.

A great book was published in 2018 titled *Estrogen Matters: Why Taking Hormones in Menopause Can Improve Women's Well-Being and Lengthen Their Lives—Without Raising the Risk of Breast Cancer.*

Authors Carol Tavris, PhD, and Avrum Bluming, MD, offer a sobering and revelatory read. *Estrogen Matters* sets the record straight on this beneficial treatment and provides an empowering path to wellness for women everywhere.[173]

I keep waiting for someone to try to show me that it's OK to have a disease. Our goal is to avoid illness. Without testosterone, there's no estrogen. The remedy offered is often to try to knock out symptoms with addictive pills that have troublesome side effects. Many problems disappear if you get hormone levels back to youthful chemistry.

Why is it wrong to stop the discomfort of aging? What's the downside of preventing dementia, stopping osteoporosis, or stopping bladder infections? "Watchful waiting" does not make any sense to me. What are you watching for? Why wait? Do you want these diseases to attack you before you put up your defenses? You could enjoy intimacy with your partner again. You might enjoy traveling healthily with a healthy partner. You might see the doctor less. Your life will have new energy.

That's all we're trying to do. That's our Holy Grail. That's our journey.

Are we willing to track you for your entire life and keep your hormones at the optimal level?

One hundred percent. Why not? You will see that restoring your youthful chemistry is like compounding interest. It grows on itself. Because now, you have more energy. You're watching your brain work; you're walking more. You astonish your friends with your youthful demeanor and body.

What other things can our hormones do? And why would we live over half of our life without them? What could we alleviate? Visceral fat, diabetes, osteoporosis, dementia, all these things if we had a youthful chemistry. I love this restoration of youth. It's the coolest thing I have ever seen. I think that's why it is vital that while we replace your diminished hormones, we're training folks to use powerful supplements like vitamins D and B12, learn how to sleep, eat, exercise, and remove stress.

> **I love this restoration of youth. It's the coolest thing I have ever seen.**

The number one cause of death in women is cardiovascular disease. Here's a way to help slow down the progress.

Dementia is significantly higher after menopause. Here's a way to attack that.

Osteoporosis is through the roof as women age.

Johns Hopkins Medicine reminds us that our body regularly replaces the components of your bones:

"When those components are lost too rapidly or not replenished quickly enough (or both), osteoporosis occurs. Osteoporosis affects more than ten million Americans. While women are at higher risk for the disease, men can develop it, too. Studies suggest that among those 50 and older:

- Up to one in two women will break a bone due to osteoporosis—equal to the risk of breast, ovarian and uterine cancer combined.

- Up to one in four men will break a bone due to osteoporosis—a risk greater than prostate cancer."[174]

In the Global Consensus Statement on Menopausal Hormone Therapy (endorsed by the American Society for Reproductive Medicine, the Asia Pacific Menopause Federation, the Endocrine Society, the European Menopause and Andropause Society, the International Menopause Society, the International Osteoporosis Foundation and the North American Menopause Society), it has been clearly stated that HRT is effective and appropriate for the prevention of osteoporosis-related fractures in at-risk women before the age of sixty years or within ten years after menopause.[175]

Because at the biochemical, cellular level, restoring hormones is a phenomenal way to make the body be its best. Therefore, we can make these phases of life more manageable.

Why in the United States does a woman have a one-in-five lifetime chance of developing dementia at age sixty-five, compared with one in nine for a man at the same age?[176]

American women live an average of five years longer than men, but "longevity does not wholly explain the higher frequency and lifetime risk," noted an expert panel representing the Society for Women's Health Research in a 2018 analysis.

In a May 1, 2020, article, the *Scientific American* asks:

- "Being female is a risk factor for Alzheimer's ... Why?

- Why are females who carry the e4 variant of the gene APOE (APOE4), which increases the risk of Alzheimer's, likely to acquire the disease at a younger age than male carriers?

- What is it about women's biology and life experiences that makes them more vulnerable?"[177]

The menopause hypothesis—that decline in estrogen levels in this period renders the brain vulnerable to future damage—could offer answers.[178]

I prepared *Restore* to convince you that hormone restoration should be in your future. All the reasons for not taking it seriously have disappeared. Let's go fill up your tank and get your twenty-five-year-old chemistry back. It's really a grand adventure! Get back into life. It's a miracle!

Look at your reflection in the lake; you're a swan. Show everyone your grace and beauty.

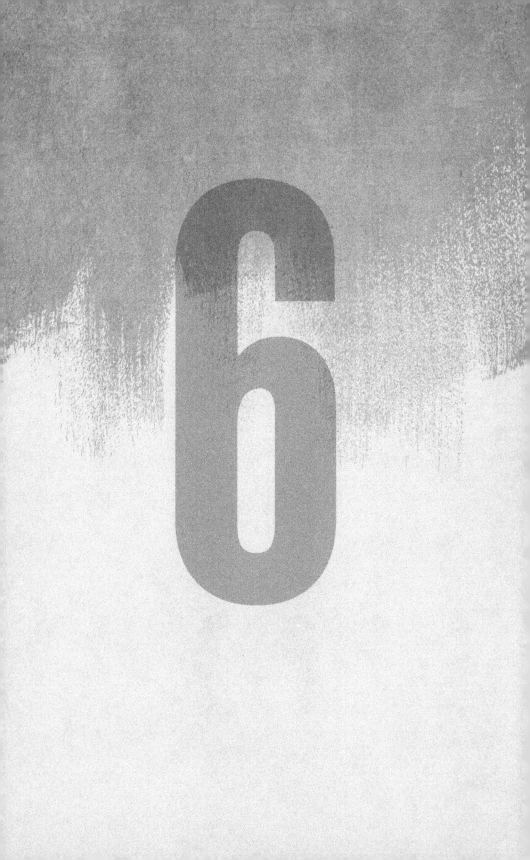

Men's Lifetime of Choices for Optimal Health—It's Much More Than Testosterone

I laugh in the face of danger.

—SIMBA, *THE LION KING*

Just picture a lion. Lions never have to tell anybody that they're a lion. It's evident. A lion never gets hyper. A lion does not try to prove itself. A lion is a lion, calm and confident. But getting to be a lion means being a cub. And being a cub means that difficulties lie ahead.

That also holds true for young boys becoming men. Hormones brew in the young male body:

- Testosterone

- Follicle-stimulating hormones (FSH) and luteinizing hormones (LH)

- Prolactin

- Estradiol

- Sex hormone-binding globulin (SHBG)

- Thyroid-stimulating hormone (TSH)

- Cortisol

PUBERTY AND ADOLESCENCE

Crucial even in the womb, testosterone determines if the genotype will be exposed as a male or female phenotype. Later in life, that's crucial for spermatogenesis, which begins a self-renewing stem cell pool. Male germ cells develop in the testes throughout life, from puberty to old age.

Testosterone provides the secondary sexual characteristics that make a man a man. It causes the musculature of the larynx to change, revealing a deeper voice, sometimes startling the puzzled parents. It changes us from cubs into lions. It also makes a woman a woman at lower levels of testosterone.

Our young cub's muscles grow. Boys take longer to mature than girls. Sexual and other physical maturation that happens during puberty results from hormonal changes. In boys, it's difficult to know exactly when puberty will arrive. Changes happen, but they occur slowly over a period of time rather than as a single event.

For 96 percent of North American males, puberty begins between 9.8 and 14.2 years, with a mean of 11.8 years (approximately two years later than girls).[179]

Changes occur over a longer period in body hair, penis, and muscle and skeletal growth. The bones of young men do not fully fuse until in the midtwenties, their muscularity in the late twenties or even early thirties.

The penis size changes as the testicles descend more. When puberty hormones increase, teenagers may have an increase in oily skin and sweating, a normal part of growing. It's important to wash daily, especially the face, to help prevent acne.

As the penis enlarges, the teen boy may begin to have erections. The penis fills with blood and becomes hard and erect. Hormones cue this, and it may happen when the boy fantasizes about sexual things. Or it may happen for no reason at all.

I'm sure my brother grew a foot between his junior and senior years in high school. The epiphyseal plates in the bone fuse because of estrogen and testosterone. They open more, so boys grow taller. Girls' estrogen levels close that plate earlier. That's why they're usually shorter because they mature sooner, corresponding to their early fertility window.

Puberty comes over a longer range because boys have more time for their bones and muscles to grow. For lion cubs, male lion manes really start to show at around the age of two years but will only become large and impressive after they reach eight years of age.[180]

At eleven months of age, they will become more adventurous, not unlike adolescent boys. As the Kariega Game Reserve in South Africa notes, they often test their folks' limits.[181]

Like the young lions, a struggle for independence and control comes with all this, as many parents know, created by the increase in testosterone. The very first thing testosterone affects is behavior. It's the brain's neuroplasticity, tweaking depression or anxiety, which happens when the testosterone levels diminish. The brain needs us to grow. Behavior is a crucial function of healthy testosterone levels, a healthy sign that *spermatogenesis has* occurred, and bone and muscle change.

On average, male fertility may happen between ages twelve and fifteen. Once the body produces mature sperm, that cues the testicles to descend. Testicles drop from the inner scrotum because our body temperature averages 98.6 degrees. Sperm matures around 94 to 96 degrees. They descend to get away from the central core heat of the body. If a *varicocele*, a vein over the testicle grows too big, it brings blood there, making it warmer. That could lower sperm count, which now reacts to temperature as well as age.

Semen, made up of sperm and other body fluids, may release during an erection, known as ejaculation. Sometimes this may happen while asleep. These wet dreams, or nocturnal emissions, represent a normal part of puberty. Once sperm is made and ejaculation happens, teen boys who have sex can get someone pregnant.

Parents of our young cubs hope and pray their kids learn right from wrong and make good decisions. That comes with maturity, and at times, kids get into trouble on the way to that lofty goal. All kids want to grow up. There's that fine line that exists between the confusion of youth and the temperance of an adult, thoughtful human being.

So wise parents become their guidepost.

Parenting gets nerve-racking because of the continuous barrage of adolescent hormones becoming a little out of whack, and they don't have the maturity yet to make good decisions.

Johns Hopkins Medicine:

WHAT DOES MY TEEN UNDERSTAND?[182]

The following are some of the abilities you may see in your teenager:

- Developing the ability to think abstractly
- Concerned with philosophy, politics, and social issues
- Thinking long term
- Setting goals
- Comparing himself to his peers

YOUR TEEN'S RELATIONSHIPS WITH OTHERS

As your teenager begins to struggle for independence and control, many changes may happen. Here are some of the issues that your teen may experience during these years:

- He wants independence from parents.
- Peer influence and acceptance are very important.
- Peer relationships become very important.
- He may be in love.
- He may have long-term commitments in relationships.

As a dad, I like to offer a very wide playing field. *Be you. Just be you.* But we must learn some things we need to avoid along the way. I do not make it so narrow that life's not fun living because I believe God wants us to find joy in life and live it abundantly and freely. I don't like being handed a thick rulebook, and neither do my kids. I understand the conflict during this change of hormones as their bodies change. I understand all that, but *don't put yourself in a position to fail.*

> **Earlier, I suggested that men have it easier than women. I think that's true, but growing from a cub into a lion is never easy.**

Consequences offer big lessons, often served with mistakes. Earlier, I suggested that men have it easier than women. I think that's true, but growing from a cub into a lion is never easy.

Young men may notice that those who mature earlier tend to become bigger risk-takers. They're like the cubs that wander too far from mom and dad too early in life, curious, willing to roll the dice a bit and see what's out there. No consideration for the consequences of that. These early maturing young men may not grow as tall as others in their age group because of that earlier growth span.

The phenomenon of male bully behavior as an adolescent eventually levels out when the early maturing bully discovers a few years later that his victims have grown bigger than him. Often, it's "apologies all around" at the reunions. I hate bullying. But I think hormones play a significant role in that thoughtless behavior.

Risk-taking can result in good or bad behavior. Risk-takers boldly go where no man has gone before. They start businesses. They explore their world. They pursue their dreams. Beneficial risky behavior can occur in a mature brain. *Start the company up, start the career, start the job, start things—what's over the mountain?* That's what you want to have. But you need to calculate the risk and benefit without encountering paralysis by analysis.

Growing from a cub to a lion is never easy.

BECOMING AN ADULT MAN: AND YOU THOUGHT GROWING UP WAS TOUGH?

By our midtwenties, men's hormones peak to optimal levels. That's a good thing because, as adults, we begin to encounter heavier and heavier loads. As in *The Lion King*, we begin to experience unforgettable lessons about life and death, depression, shame, envy, betrayal, friendship, greed, respect, desperation, fear, leadership, sibling rivalry, love, devastation, forgiving yourself, and even marrying your best friend![183]

Testosterone helps you deal with all this. This hormone first helps with behavior early in adolescence. Usually, it kicks in fully as we become young men, helping the immune system, the brain, bone, muscle, heart, and other hormones. It protects against diabetes, heart issues, cancer, and the entire immune system. It helps prostate health.

A crusading knight mounting his horse comes to mind, preparing for a life of watchful protection of the pilgrims, perhaps squired by a son, who serves as shield carrier and assists in preparing for the journey, or for battle.

The twenties also introduce us to the beginnings of metabolic syndrome, a cluster of conditions that occur together, increasing your risk of heart disease, stroke, and type 2 diabetes. These conditions include increased blood pressure, high blood sugar, excess body fat around the waist, and abnormal cholesterol or triglyceride levels.[184]

We either wake up to healthy lifestyle choices or bear the slings and arrows of outrageous fortune.

Young Guys with Older-Guy Problems

We see more and more men and women in their twenties, which now represent about 25 percent of our patients, and they arrive in our office with the same complaints as fifty-year-olds. When your hormones are not at their optimal level, what do you have? Behavior disorders, weak muscles, increased atherosclerosis, belly fat, erection problems, brain fog, poor libido, anxiety, lack of energy, and maybe depression. You have all of those because the body does not have the optimal fuel, and that's the problem. What does testosterone do? Oh, it's part of everything. So what happens if you lose it? You lose part of everything.

We're probably not to blame. The environment has a lot to say about our hormone health. If we can keep our hormone levels in the optimal range, then we'd have fewer adrenal problems, fewer stress problems, and fewer side effects of all that. Testosterone, I believe, goes down with age, not because of age, but because of the accumulated time you spend living in this sick environment amid all the neuroendocrine disruptors, the *xenoestrogens*. In the not-too-distant future, we will look back and say, "How in the world did we allow this pollution?"

Hormones are chemical messengers created by the body to transfer information from one set of cells to another. As hormones are released into the bloodstream, they coordinate and control the various functions of the body to maintain health and stability. The endocrine system in your body is made up of glands that produce and secrete hormones to regulate the activity of cells or organs. Hormones regulate the body's growth, metabolism, sexual development, and function. When our hormone levels drop, becoming unbalanced, our health is affected. The hormones created and released by the glands in your body's endocrine system control nearly all the processes in your body. These chemicals help coordinate your body's functions, from metabolism to growth and development, emotions, mood, sexual function and even sleep.

As we have shown, hormones are chemicals that coordinate different functions in your body by carrying messages through your blood to your organs, skin, muscles, and other tissues. These signals tell your body what to do and when to do it. Sometimes your endocrine glands produce too much or not enough of a hormone. This imbalance can cause health problems, such as weight gain, high blood pressure and changes in sleep, mood, and behavior. Many things can affect how your body creates and releases hormones. Illness, stress, and certain medications can cause a hormone imbalance. For men, some of the most common disorders are diabetes, thyroid disease, low testosterone (low T), and osteoporosis. Endocrine disruptors can also affect hormone balance. These chemicals appear everywhere—in pesticides, plastics, cosmetics and even our food and water.

When chemicals from the outside get into our bodies, they have the ability to mimic our natural hormones. The invaders block or bind hormone receptors, detrimental to hormone-sensitive organs like the uterus and the breast, the immune and neurological systems, as well as general human development.

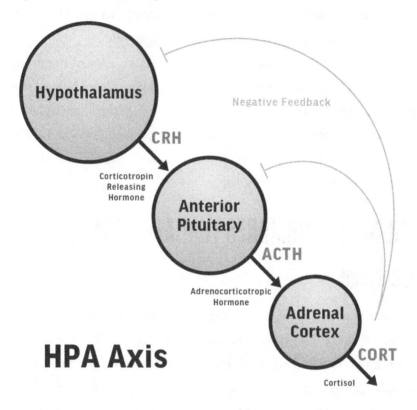

For your entire life, your body has been bombarded by these chemicals that lower testosterone. The only hormone that increases with age is cortisol. Older men *should* have relatively the same amount of testosterone as younger men, but clearly that is not the case today. Cortisol goes up with age, and that creates havoc and stress in the body.

Recall that testosterone's very first impact other than sexual characteristics is behavior. I see twenty-five-to-thirty-year-old young men coming in with a list of complaints: brain fog, no motivation, weak erections, and lack of energy. It drives me crazy. The problem drives the behavior, first and foremost. If primary care providers don't even question hormone levels that early in life, they're dead wrong. Many do not question low testosterone because these guys live in the "wrong age group." But they're reacting to the wrong assumptions. Why would you not look at the fuel that makes this behavior? Why not test for testosterone or a vitamin D deficiency?

When young men like these come in, I ask a lot of questions. How's your diet? How's your exercise? How's your sleep? What drugs do you take? Do you augment your reality with virtual games? Many have not shed their teenage habits, and the gamble is now due. They once knew, but have forgotten, how to be a man. They have disassociated themselves from that as well.

THE SEVEN HORMONES THAT AFFECT MEN
1. Cortisol

Though widely known as the body's stress hormone, Cortisol has a variety of effects on different functions throughout the body. It is the main glucocorticoid released from the zona fasciculata, the middle zone of the adrenal cortex. The hypothalamus-pituitary-adrenal axis regulates both production and secretion of cortisol. Loss of regulation can lead to cortisol excess disorders, such as Cushing syndrome, or cortical insufficiency, such as Addison disease.

Cortisol, a steroid hormone, is synthesized from cholesterol. The body's regulation of cortisol is critical. Here's how it is achieved: it is synthesized in the zona fasciculata layer of the adrenal cortex. Adrenocorticotropic hormone (ACTH), released from the anterior pituitary, functions to increase LDL receptors and increase the activity of cholesterol desmolase, which converts cholesterol to pregnenolone and is the rate-limiting step of cortisol synthesis. Cortisol is a steroid in the same class as estrogen, testosterone, and progesterone.

Blood levels of cortisol vary throughout the day, but generally are higher in the morning when we wake up, and then fall throughout the day, and we call that a diurnal rhythm. In people that work at night, this pattern is reversed. The timing of cortisol release is clearly linked to daily activity.

In addition, in response to stress, extra cortisol is released to help the body to respond appropriately. Endocrine glands on top of your kidneys produce and release cortisol, which affects several aspects of your body and mainly helps regulate your body's response to stress. It owes its existence to cholesterol. Cholesterol's four rings eventually produce pregnenolone. Cortisol comes from that chain reaction, becoming a response hormone, which creates a rapid increase in sugar and a rapid increase of beta-oxidation of fat. Make energy, *flight or fight.*

Too little cortisol may be caused by a problem in the pituitary gland or the adrenal gland (Addison's disease). The onset of symptoms is often very gradual. Symptoms may include fatigue, dizziness (especially when standing), weight loss, muscle weakness, mood changes, and the darkening of regions of the skin. Without treatment, this is a potentially life-threatening condition.

The Controversy around Cholesterol and Statins

Fifty percent of all people who experience a heart attack have normal cholesterol.[185]

Cholesterol is essential for:

- Formation and maintenance of cell membranes (essential for life)

- Making hormones such as progesterone testosterone, estradiol, and cortisol

- Production of bile salts, which help to digest food

- Conversion of sunlight into vitamin D in the skin

Our cells need cholesterol to thrive—including those in your brain. Mood disorders can be seen when the cholesterol is too low.

We get approximately one-third of our cholesterol from what we eat. Two-thirds of cholesterol is made by the liver. Very low cholesterol may mean your body is shutting down and unable to make its own cholesterol.

TIME magazine reports that the US Centers for Disease Control and Prevention (CDC) notes that about 93 million American adults have high cholesterol, which represents about 36 percent of the US adult population.[186]

TIME also reported that according to the CDC, statin use has been growing for the past decade, and nearly 39 million Americans take a statin daily. Usage increases over age forty since heart risks tend to escalate as we get older.[187]

Side effects can concern folks. The major complaint seems to be myopathy, a neuromuscular disorder that causes muscle pain. Statin-associated muscle symptoms can include mild-to-moderate pain, fatigue, weakness, and night cramps.

Are you confused about cholesterol and the need for stains?

Mirroring the CDC report, about 40 million adults in the United States regularly take statins to lower their cholesterol levels and reduce their risk of heart disease and stroke, according to American Heart Association data from 2020.[188]

However, many of them don't stand to benefit from these drugs based on new research from Dr. David Diamond, a University of South Florida neuroscientist and cardiovascular disease researcher in the Department of Psychology.[189]

The University of South Florida Newsroom reported on September 19, 2022, that Dr. Diamond and his coauthors reviewed literature from medical trials involving patients taking either a statin or placebo. They then narrowed their review to look at study participants with elevated levels of low-density lipoprotein-cholesterol (LDL), the so-called "bad cholesterol," which can be reduced with a statin.

"Some individuals with high LDL also had high triglycerides (fat in the blood) and low high-density lipoprotein (HDL), the 'good cholesterol,' which put them at the highest risk of having a heart attack," the USF publication noted.

"But others with high LDL were very different. They had low triglycerides and high HDL, which meant they were healthier. People with optimal triglycerides and HDL levels typically exercise, have low blood pressure and low blood sugar, and are at a low risk of a heart attack."[190]

"Their findings, published in the journal *Current Opinion in Endocrinology, Diabetes and Obesity*, showed LDL alone has 'a very weak association' with heart disease and stroke. Their review went further, showing that when people with high LDL and optimal triglycerides and HDL were given a statin, there was no benefit." [191]

Dr. Diamond concluded, "Our findings show that the people who have this healthy combination of diet and lifestyle, as well as high LDL, showed no benefit from taking a statin. "[192]

The USF publication also noted that Dr. Diamond acknowledges that his research is controversial and has resulted in strong support, along with criticism from some within the medical community who have challenged his views on LDL and statins. He cautions that it is intended to raise awareness and should not be considered medical advice.[193]

The association of cardiovascular diseases is not "total cholesterol." The association is the particle number, the leading indicator of inflammation. Cardiovascular disease, at its root cause, is an inflammatory response. So it's not total cholesterol or LDL, but it's particle number. That increases oxidative stress, which leads to inflammatory response and can cause atherosclerosis.

Health Matters notes that traditional lipid testing "measures the amount of LDL cholesterol (LDL-C) present in the blood, but it does not evaluate the number of LDL particles (LDL-P)."

"LDL-P is often used to get a more accurate measure of LDL due to the variability of cholesterol content within a given LDL. Studies have shown that LDL-P more accurately predicts risk of cardiovascular disease than LDL-C," notes the Health Matters website to help folks interpret their lab reports.

"Researchers think that increased LDL-P could be one of the reasons that some people have heart attacks even though their total cholesterol and LDL cholesterol levels are not particularly high."[194]

As always, learn all you can; make your own decision.

2. Thyroid-Stimulating Hormone (TSH)

Thyroid-stimulating hormone (TSH) is a hormone that your pituitary gland releases to trigger your thyroid to produce and release its own hormones—T4 thyroxine, T3 triiodothyronine, and reverse T3. These three hormones maintain your body's metabolic rate—the speed at which your body transforms the food you eat into energy and uses it. Thyroxine and triiodothyronine also maintain heart, brain, bone, and muscle functions.

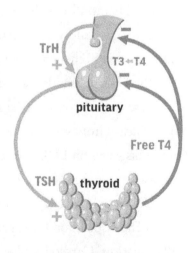

Picture a bow tie in your neck, and that it makes four hormones you know about (T1, T2, T3, T4), all based upon how many iodine molecules it has on that structure.

3. Estradiol

Estradiol (E2) is an estrogen steroid hormone and the major female sex hormone. Though at much lower levels than in females, estradiol has important roles in males as well. There are four estrogens—estrone (E1), estradiol (E2) estriol (E3), and estetrol (E4)—involved in the regulation of the estrous and menstrual female reproductive cycles. Estradiol is responsible for the development of female secondary sexual character-istics such as the breasts, widening of the hips, and a female-associated pattern of fat distribution. It also has important effects in many other tissues, including bone, fat, skin, liver, and the brain. With testosterone, it becomes estrogen with aromatase. Estrogen keeps the arteries relaxed and lowers blood pressure. It helps the blood flow better to the penis, the heart, and the brain. Too high and we have a mood problem, too low and we encounter erection problems. There's a sweet spot in there, and it helps make the cardiovascular system and the brain optimal. Men need it for brain and cardiovascular protection.

4. Prolactin

Prolactin is a hormone that's responsible for lactation, certain breast tissue development and contributes to hundreds of other bodily processes. Prolactin levels, normally low in males and nonlactating and nonpregnant people, come from your pituitary gland. It makes and releases (secretes) the hormone. Prolactin helps intimacy and mood. It's made back to the hypothalamus again. It has a thing called prolactin-releasing hormone that releases a hormone from the angio pituitary. I check prolactin and LH in every single man before they get started with hormone replacement. Why? Being watchful for prolactinoma.

A prolactinoma is not life-threatening, but it can cause vision difficulties, infertility, and other problems. Prolactinoma is the most common type of hormone-producing tumor that can develop in the pituitary gland, but it should not be left untreated because a prolactinoma can cause reduced hormone production if the tumor presses on the pituitary gland, which may lead to weight loss or fatigue, possibly osteoporosis (brittle, fragile bones) or pregnancy complications.

5. FSH and LH

Follicle-stimulating hormone (FSH) stimulates sperm production. Then on the other side of the brain, the luteinizing hormone (LH) produces testosterone, which then converts to estradiol and dihydrotestosterone, five to ten times more potent than testosterone. Their main function in this setting is to mature sperm. FSH plays an important role in sexual development and functioning. Too much or too little FSH can cause various problems, including infertility, menstrual difficulties in women, low sex drive in men, and early or delayed puberty in children.

6. Testosterone

The testes synthesize two essential products: testosterone, needed for the development and maintenance of many physiological functions, including normal testis function; and sperm, required for male fertility. The synthesis of both products is regulated by endocrine hormones produced in the hypothalamus and pituitary, as well as locally within the testis.[195]

7. Testosterone and Sperm Production

The secretion of hypothalamic gonadotropin-releasing hormone (GnRH) stimulates the production of luteinizing hormone (LH) and follicle stimulating hormone (FSH) by the pituitary.

LH is transported in the bloodstream to the testes, where it stimulates Leydig cells to produce testosterone: this can act as an androgen (via interaction with androgen receptors) but can also be aromatized to produce estrogens.

The testes give feedback on the hypothalamus and the pituitary via testosterone and inhibin secretion in a negative feedback loop to limit GnRH and gonadotropin production.

Both androgens and FSH act on receptors within the supporting somatic cells, the Sertoli cells, to stimulate various functions needed for optimal sperm production:

Spermatogenesis is the process by which immature male germ cells divide, undergo meiosis, and differentiate into highly specialized haploid spermatozoa. Optimal spermatogenesis requires the action of both testosterone (via androgen receptors) and FSH. Androstenedione, a steroid hormone, increases the production of the hormone testosterone, which enhances athletic performance, builds muscle, reduces body fat, increases energy, keeps red blood cells healthy, increases sexual desire and performance, and mellows behavior. This is a powerful hormone in both men and women.[196]

HIGH GLUCOSE AND HIGH INSULIN: THE CULPRITS THAT CAN THROW ALL THIS OFF

High glucose and insulin can become the culprits for throwing all this off because they can act in the brain as neurotransmitters and cause the connection to misfire. Plus, they could bind glucose and fructose, which distorts their structure and function. That's what we call Alzheimer's now, unofficially dubbed "type 3 diabetes." When they're not being produced at proper levels, bad things happen.

If we can keep our hormone levels in the optimal range, then we'll have fewer chronic disease problems. We inhale toxic pesticide fumes, breathe pollutants in the air and water, and leech mercury amalgam fillings in our mouths. We're exposed to tobacco smoke, asbestos, plastic, and all the by-now-well-known things that can kill us in everyday life, the nasty neuroendocrine disruptors, the *xenoestrogens*. The Women's Health Network describes the scope of this at-times invisible threat:

More than 80,000 chemicals have been registered with the EPA since World War II, with at least 2,000 new ones added annually in the US alone, and it's not slowing down. We're all vulnerable to toxic exposure, including children. PCBs and DDT have been detected, for example, in 50 percent and 70 percent, respectively, of kids as young as four years old. The glowing promise of "better living through chemistry" has tragically backfired as pollution intensifies and its associated health hazards become more apparent.[197]

LOW T BROADCAST COMMERCIALS

We have all seen and heard the annoying radio and television commercials promoting low T remedies. Why has an entire industry sprung up to help men with their libido and to achieve noble erections? I would venture to guess that over half of the adult population of young men over thirty seeks or contemplates seeking such a remedy. Men clearly willing to pay hundreds of dollars for a few blue pills will try anything that may relieve their symptoms. They're too young for that, and I agree 100 percent with their doing something about it. I have a problem with these remedies. They work for a while and provide welcome relief, but they do not address the invisible cause, the inevitable-but-way-too-early loss of hormones.[198]

GRADUAL HORMONAL DECLINE
of TESTOSTERONE *in male body*

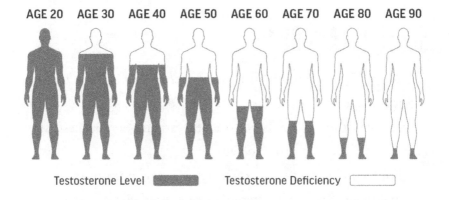

Medanta, "Patient education: Signs you are experiencing hormone imbalance," https://www.medanta.org/patient-education-blog/signs-youre-experiencing-a-hormone-imbalance-for-men/, accessed January 22, 2023.

This chart, created by Medanta, the largest private hospital in India, illustrates worldwide concerns about declining testosterone levels.

These disruptors affect testosterone all over the planet. Our developing world culture has experienced a population-wide catastrophic decline in testosterone levels that began fifty years ago.

We can point the finger at our food consumption. We're seeing scary increases in diabetes, central obesity, and high blood pressure. We inherited all this because of this crazy American diet they gave us, this now-disavowed 1977 food pyramid that got us away from proper nutrition. The United States Department of Agriculture (USDA) created the food pyramid. It placed grains at the base of the pyramid (eat all the bread you can), with veggies and fruits on the next largest tier.

They championed foods to comprise most of our three-meal-a-day diets. We should change our then-high-fat-high protein diet, they said, and we should eat low fat, low protein, and imbibe all the carbohydrates we can find.

A lot can go wrong if our lifestyle becomes unhealthy.

ADRENAL FATIGUE

The Mayo Clinic reminds us that *adrenal fatigue* isn't an accepted medical diagnosis. It is a lay term applied to a collection of non-specific symptoms, such as body aches, fatigue, nervousness, sleep disturbances and digestive problems.[199]

Your adrenal glands produce a variety of hormones that are essential to life. The medical term "adrenal insufficiency" refers to the inadequate production of one or more of these hormones as a result of an underlying disease or surgery.

Signs and symptoms of adrenal insufficiency may include:

- Fatigue

- Body aches

- Unexplained weight loss

- Low blood pressure

- Lightheadedness

- Loss of body hair

- Skin discoloration (hyperpigmentation)

Adrenal insufficiency can be diagnosed by blood tests and special stimulation tests that show inadequate levels of adrenal hormones.

Landmark Study Defines Normal Ranges for Testosterone Levels

*New defined reference range can help limit misdiagnoses and unnecessary treatments,
January 10, 2017*

The Journal of Clinical Endocrinology & Metabolism of the Endocrine Society announrge study of more than nine thousand men has established harmonized reference ranges for total testosterone in men. When applied to assays that have been appropriately calibrated, this will effectively enable clinicians to make a correct diagnosis of hypogonadism. according to the journal.

The study, "Harmonized Reference Ranges for Circulating Testosterone Levels in Men of Four Cohort Studies in the USA and Europe," is designed to help the correct diagnosis and effective treatment and prevention of hypogonadism as well as many other diseases, which depend on accurate measurement of hormones, but lack of both defined reference ranges of testosterone and standardization of hormone assays has made diagnosing hypogonadism a difficult task.

"Well-defined reference ranges are at the heart of clinical practice and without them clinicians can make erroneous diagnoses that could lead to patients receiving costly, lifelong treatments that they don't need or deny treatments to those who need them," said Shalender Bhasin, MD, of Brigham and Women's Hospital, Harvard Medical School in Boston, and lead author of the study. "Clearly, we need standardization in all hormone assays."[337]

The harmonized normal range for testosterone in a nonobese population of European and American Men, nineteen to thirty-nine years, is 264–916 ng/dL.[338] As an example, let's look back five years at the ranges. Five years ago, the 2017 levels were published as 348–1,197. Significantly higher, begging the question: Why are the reference ranges being regularly lowered?

Mayo Clinic adds:

> Proponents of the adrenal fatigue diagnosis claim this is
> a mild form of adrenal insufficiency caused by chronic
> stress. The unproven theory behind adrenal fatigue is
> that your adrenal glands are unable to keep pace with
> the demands of perpetual fight-or-flight arousal. Existing
> blood tests, according to this theory, aren't sensitive
> enough to detect such a small decline in adrenal function—
> but your body is.[200]

Normal levels heighten memory, enhance your immune system, regulate body sugar levels and blood pressure, and even strengthen the heart. But stress fires it up. While it's kept us alive for eons, it represents a double-edged sword.

As cortisol rallies a response to danger, *flight or fight*, it goes up for seconds to minutes at a time. Our Western world stays chronically elevated because of continuous stresses: the computers, the video, corporate worry, financial pressures, even the news. But if your thyroid stays in balance, your testosterone, estrogen, and progesterone will take response pressure off the adrenals. As cortisol scores go up, the stressful environment impacts youthful chemistry.

I have a four-step protocol on adrenals. We use simple saliva tests. We can check cortisol with saliva because saliva gives us an accurate number very easily and inexpensively. We track the results and create a curve. It's not just one result at a given point in time. Based on the curve of cortisol, we can stage your problem and then fine-tune the treatment.

Your adrenals, that short-term response hormone, can, in the short-term, save your life. Long term, it can make you chronically ill.

YOUR THYROID

The thyroid endocrine gland, shaped like a butterfly, resides in the lower front of the neck below the larynx (the voice box). The thyroid makes thyroid hormones, secreted into the blood, and then carried to every tissue in the body.

The thyroid hormone helps the body use energy, stay warm and keep the brain, heart, muscles, and other organs working as they should. The main hormone made by the thyroid is thyroxine, also called T4 because it contains four iodine atoms. Small amounts of another and more potent thyroid hormone containing three iodine atoms, triiodothyronine (T3), also made by the thyroid gland. However, most of the T3 and reverse T3 in the blood is made from T4.[201]

Thyroid hormones control the way every tissue in your body uses energy, essential to help each cell in your body's tissue and organs work right. For example, the thyroid hormone controls the body's temperature, heart rate, blood pressure, and the rate at which food turns into energy (metabolism).

If you have hypothyroidism, that means you have an underactive thyroid ("hypo-" means "under" or "below normal"). In people with hypothyroidism, the thyroid does not make enough thyroid hormone to keep the body running normally. Low thyroid hormone levels cause our body's functions to slow, leading to general symptoms like dry skin, fatigue, loss of energy, and memory problems. We can diagnose hypothyroidism by simple thyroid functioning (TFH) blood tests.

Hyperthyroidism can threaten your life. Hyperthyroidism happens when the thyroid gland makes too much thyroid hormone, a condition called overactive thyroid. Hyperthyroidism speeds up the body's metabolism. That can cause many symptoms, such as weight loss, hand tremors, and rapid or irregular heartbeat.

The Mayo Clinic observes that older adults may have elusive symptoms. These symptoms may include an irregular heartbeat, weight loss, depression, and feeling weak or tired during ordinary activities.[202]

ANDROPAUSE

Male menopause is 100 percent real. It announces itself with belly fat, tiredness, brain fog, no libido, and unhealthy erections.

Again, let's look at age. Andropause kicks in because of your age? Maybe. But why does it happen with age? Because the testicles make less over time? Maybe. But maybe the toxic environment speeds that up. And that is my hypothesis. We see younger and younger men with andropause symptoms. Clinical literature varies on the age range, but I see reports that male menopause affects about 20 percent of men over age sixty and 30 to 50 percent of men over age eighty. I disagree.

When men come in, and we sit down and talk about their symptoms, the thing we expect to hear is tiredness and brain fog. We hear that a lot. We probe a bit deeper, revealing a whole spectrum of symptoms. We have a midlife crisis in that our midlife men delude themselves that they could not possibly experience male menopause.

The symptoms might include the following:

- Decrease in muscle mass and overall strength

- Decrease in bone mineral density and a corresponding increased risk of osteoporosis

- Low libido and erectile dysfunction

- Decreased energy and depression

- Cognitive impairment

Low Testosterone Levels Were Associated with an Increased Mortality Risk 88 Percent Greater Than for Men with Normal Testosterone Levels[203]

Journal of the American Medical Association
August 14, 2006

In this study of male veterans forty years and older, without prostate cancer, followed up for a mean of 4.3 years, men with low and equivocal serum testosterone levels had increased all-cause mortality and shorter survival times compared with men with normal testosterone levels.[204]

In an unadjusted model, low testosterone levels were associated with an increased mortality risk of 88 percent greater than that for men with normal testosterone levels.[205]

In the fully adjusted model, which included the covariates of age, medical morbidity, BMI (body mass index), race, and other clinical factors, low testosterone level continued to be associated with an increased mortality risk of 88 percent greater than in men with normal testosterone levels.[206]

Men experiencing any of these symptoms should ask their primary care physician or geriatrician about having testosterone levels tested, and men should start bone-density tests at age seventy or earlier if they are not on BHRT. That test may show that they indeed need hormone replacement.

A healthy lifestyle with regular exercise and a balanced diet is a part of the fight against symptoms of andropause as for menopause. You have to work a little, and there's no magic bullet. But simple changes can help with almost every symptom, but there is no substitute for bioidentical hormone replacement.

When I began writing this book, I looked for the best metaphor I could find for this age-old quest to apply the wisdom of age to age youthfully. I began to develop this idea by focusing on the search for the Holy Grail, the Knights Templar, and the courageous protection of pilgrims heading to the Holy Land.

They were religious soldiers known for their loyalty to their king, purity of heart, and phenomenal skills in combat. They were among the first to seek a remedy for the frailty of aging.

When I reached this point in our narrative, I thought of several modern-day knights I have cared for over the years and how bioidentical hormone restoration changed their lives. We see astounding responses to BHRT with veterans suffering from traumatic brain injuries and PTSD.

OUR THIRTIES AND FORTIES: THE AWAKENING

The health awakening in most men happens from the midthirties to the early forties. Realization takes hold. We start to deteriorate then and continue to deteriorate until we pass away if we do nothing about it.

I am guilty on all counts of that. In August 1996, our family enjoyed a vacation up in the mountains. I was thirty-six years old, and two things happened. I played racquetball with my older daughter and my son, and ended up unbelievably spent. Exhausted. Then, I could not fit into my dress pants for dinner. That's embarrassing. I had to buy more oversize waist pants. I had not been eating properly.

So I responded to these two catastrophes with my awakening. It took a while to figure it all out. As everyone knows, it is tough to make major lifestyle changes at the peak of your career and commitments. I started working out harder and did see early results. But it took another twelve years to really get it. No kidding. That's when I learned about the effectiveness of intermittent fasting and reducing my dependence on carbohydrates. I did the treadmill harder and harder. I ate multiple small meals a day, a highly complex carbohydrate diet. I got stronger, but I weighed in at 180 pounds. So with intermittent fasting (more in chapter 8 on nutrition), my waist reduced to thirty-two inches. I wished I had not tossed my mountain-trip pants version of myself.

By the time I turned fifty, I learned to eat properly, and my waist went down to thirty inches, and combining that with some better-planned exercise, I weighed in at 145 pounds, the top end of the *super lightweight* class in professional boxing. When I added bioidentical hormone replacement therapy to all this, my muscular structure took me back to 170 pounds, now a *super middleweight,* and my waist stayed at thirty inches. *Boom.* It all finally came together.

The Mayo Clinic offers a bit of advice for older men as regards keeping a healthy sex life:

- Take care of yourself, and stay as healthy as you can.

- Eat a healthy diet.

- Exercise regularly.

- Don't drink too much alcohol.

- Don't smoke.

- Think positive.

- Practice gratitude.

- Drink plenty of water.

- Get enough sleep.

- Make time for loved ones and hobbies.[207]

"WHEN I'M SIXTY-FOUR"
—The Beatles

When I get older losing my hair
Many years from now
Will you still be sending me a Valentine
Birthday greetings bottle of wine[208]

Well, our government and its healthcare system won't send you a valentine.

They might encourage you to get your PSA test, a blood test that has been proven ill-advised. Years after the PSA test was elbowed aside around the world, US doctors still call for the test as you get older. Perhaps they think that if they do not offer this test, they will have the risk of malpractice. Perhaps because it often calls for a needle biopsy, which gives the trusted healer a clear picture of the prostate condition. The government hasn't said one way or another about this controversial practice.

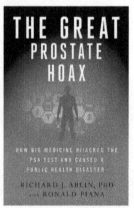

Ablin, Richard J., and Ronald Piana. *The Great Prostate Hoax: How Big Medicine Hijacked the PSA Test and Caused a Public Health Disaster.* New York, NY: St. Martin's Press, 2014.

The Great Prostate Hoax

Prostate cancer screening remains one of the most controversial clinical and public health topics. Despite being the second most common cancer in men worldwide, recommendations for screening using prostate-specific antigen (PSA) are unclear.[209]

Research Shows Men with Low Testosterone Are More Likely to Die from COVID-19

July 30, 2021

Men with symptomatic COVID-19, found to have low testosterone following admittance to the hospital, were more likely to become severely ill and die from the disease, new research has shown.

The study, carried out in Milan during the first wave of coronavirus in 2020, found that the lower the levels of testosterone, the higher the likelihood that male patients would need intensive care, intubation on a ventilator, and remain in hospital over a longer period. Their likelihood of dying increased six-fold.

The findings were presented at the 2021 European Association of Urology Congress.[210]

Over time, evidence accumulated indicating that PSA testing could lead to overdiagnosis, thus unnecessarily subjecting men to the harms of treatment. Why would you get in line for a painful and expensive needle biopsy and pay for a test of your prostate that every country in the world has deemed ineffective? Why would you endure a needle biopsy because you scored over 4 on a test that does not work? Why can't we learn? We have learned one thing for sure. Your prostate gets healthier with optimal levels of testosterone and estrogen.

If your cholesterol goes up, that's the first thing you'll hear: *here is your prescription for a statin.* Physicians often prescribe this remedy for high cholesterol.

Recent studies have raised concerns, and some suspect these powerful drugs may have a link to increased incidence of Alzheimer's and other chronic diseases. Side effects of statin therapy can "include new-onset type 2 diabetes mellitus, neurological and neurocognitive effects, hepatotoxicity, renal toxicity, and other conditions. Currently, no universally accepted definition of statin toxicity/intolerance exists."[211]

When you sign up for Medicare, here comes a flurry of telephone calls, texts, and letters suggesting that *Medicare Advantage* programs would like you to give up your choice of medical providers in exchange for a list of benefits. The volume of television commercials rivals a political campaign. It's the most obvious appeal I have ever seen in this country to voluntarily give up your medical freedom and hand over your health decisions to a team of bureaucrats. And our government applauds it.

Dr. Elizabeth Rosenthal deeply explores the subject of the medical-industrial complex in *An American Sickness: How Healthcare Became Big Business and How You Can Take It Back*, the 2017 *NPR* and *Wall Street Journal* Book of the Year and *New York Times* bestseller. The PSA issue arises among other major healthcare crises that our healthcare system has spawned in recent years.

Elisabeth Rosenthal worked as an emergency room physician before becoming a journalist. A former *New York Times* correspondent, she today serves as the editor in chief of *Kaiser Health News*. Here's the synopsis of her book:

> In these troubled times, perhaps no institution has unraveled more quickly and more completely than American medicine. In only a few decades, the medical system has been overrun by organizations seeking to exploit for profit the trust that vulnerable and sick Americans place in their healthcare. Our politicians have proven themselves either unwilling or incapable of reining in the increasingly outrageous costs

> faced by patients, and market-based solutions only seem to
> funnel larger and larger sums of our money into the hands
> of corporations. Impossibly high insurance premiums and
> inexplicably large bills have become facts of life; fatalism
> has set in. Very quickly Americans have been made to accept
> paying more for less. How did things get so bad so fast?[212]

Do your research well before you pass the age of fifty. Consider BHRT as soon as possible, and read Elizabeth Rosenthal's book *An American Sickness: How Healthcare Became Big Business and How You Can Take It Back* to better understand the crossroads ahead.

HOPE OVER 50

Family life, an important aspect of our life as we grow older, seems to represent a key to the health of older men. For years, study after study has shown a correlation between a lack of social support and a higher risk of mortality. Supportive relationships are associated with lower illness rates, faster recovery rates, and better attention to health.

So much can go wrong because of the loss of hormones, it blows the mind. In our episodic-sick-care-designed medical marketplace, your provider may not recognize that and start to treat these troubling symptoms of anxiety, moods, libido, and aging with unnecessary and harmful drugs, or, worse, therapies and surgical interventions that could have been prevented.

We have been hammered from the womb and clinicians still call that *normal*. We can fix your hormone depletion. We can resolve these complaints and create a new day of youthful wellness and aging now. If you do not act to replace your hormones, you're missing the first chance in history to confidently do something about that. Look around you. Here's what we may see as men start becoming frail:

- Fatigue

- Cognitive function decline

- Decreased libido

- Erectile dysfunction

- Depression

- Irritability

- Decreased sense of well-being

- Decreased muscle mass

- Increased body fat

- Decreased bone mineral density

The Mayo Clinic reports:

> Recommendations on testosterone therapy for men with age-related low testosterone vary. In 2020, the American College of Physicians recommended that doctors consider starting testosterone treatment in men with sexual dysfunction who want to improve their sexual function, after explaining the risks and benefits. In 2018, the Endocrine Society recommended testosterone therapy for men with age-related low testosterone who have signs and symptoms associated with low testosterone.[213]

My knowledge speaks loudly to me to begin bioidentical hormone replacement as soon as the symptoms appear. I will not use the term "age-related."

If you become an eighty-year-old lion, most of all of that will disappear. And I'll bet you have less diabetes, less osteoporosis, less prostate cancer, less breast cancer, fewer heart issues, and less belly

For Older Adults, "Hope" May Be a Key Piece for Improving Health, Psychological, and Social Well-Being

Virginia Commonwealth University News, February 14, 2020[328]

Older adults with a greater sense of hope have a better likelihood of experiencing good physical health outcomes and better psychological and social well-being, according to a new study.[329]

The study, "The role of *hope* in subsequent health and well-being for older adults: An outcome-wide longitudinal approach," was led by researchers affiliated with the Human Flourishing Program at Harvard University's Institute for Quantitative Social Science and coauthored by Everett Worthington, PhD, emeritus Commonwealth professor in the Department of Psychology in VCU's College of Humanities and Sciences.[330]

The researchers analyzed data on nearly thirteen thousand older adults in the Health and Retirement Study, a longitudinal and nationally representative data set of adults over age fifty. They found that a greater sense of hope associated with better physical health and health behavior outcomes on some indicators (such as fewer chronic conditions, a lower risk of cancer, and fewer sleep problems), higher psychological well-being (such as greater life satisfaction and purpose in life), lower psychological distress, and better social well-being.[331]

Dr. Worthington recently discussed the study, which he says may hold important implications for improving the physical, psychological, and social health of the United States' growing older adult population: "Hope gives people meaning. It yields a more positive mood; fewer mental health symptoms; more healthy exercise, eating and weight; more powerful self-control; more social engagement with family and friends; and practice of religion in religious communities."[332]

> **Because we have the youth of a young lion and the maturity of an eighty-year-old lion, we have found the sweet spot. That's the key. That's what we're trying to do here.**

fat. Because we have the youth of a young lion and the maturity of an eighty-year-old lion, we have found the sweet spot. That's the key. That's what we're trying to do here. We applaud maturity but urge you to have your cells at the optimal metabolic level to benefit from your wisdom.

It's the circle of life, and it moves us all, through despair and hope, through faith and love, till we find our place, on the path unwinding.

—ELTON JOHN

Lawlinguists offers more interesting observations about the worldwide power and meaning of the lyrics of *The Lion King*:

The opening song of *The Lion King* has some pretty distinctive lyrics, though few of us actually know what all of them mean. "The Circle of Life" starts out in Zulu before switching over to English. Here are the immortal words of Elton John, Tim Rice, and the animals of the Savannah:

> *Nants ingonyama bagithi Baba*
> *Sithi uhm ingonyama*
> *Nants ingonyama bagithi baba*
> *Sithi uhhmm ingonyama*
> *Ingonyama*
> *Siyo Nqoba*
> *Ingonyama*
> *Ingonyama nengw' enamabala.*

If you speak Zulu, it might be pretty underwhelming. But those who aren't fluent in the language have likely never understood those

Hope and optimism are different, Dr. Worthington explains: "*Optimism* suggests being positive about outcomes. *Hope*, however, does not mean that the outcome will be positive, but it keeps people engaged and moving forward," he said.[333]

Hope has three parts: *willpower* to change, *waypower* to change, and *waitpower* when we don't see change happening. As people age, we can see a definite shift in the type of hope they experience.

"At 30, the world is in front of us at our feet. We mostly experience hope as a sense of agency (i.e., that I can affect change) and pathways (i.e., I have lots of ways to change things, so I must stay resilient to use the right strategy at the right time)," he adds.[334]

When people in their thirties to early sixties encounter hardships, it's mostly about external barriers that keep getting in their paths. So resilience pathways help to maintain hope that keeps people striving toward their goals. Dr. Worthington explained that in older people—and this study started with people aged sixty-six and looked at them over time—many of the obstacles seem insolvable. They encounter health challenges that may not heal.[335]

"There are losses of significant people. There are collapses in social networks, especially as people retire and might lose functioning and experience impaired mobility and freedom," he noted.

The researchers observed that we need the type of hope that allows us to persevere even when they do not think they can overcome the challenges.

Good strategies include cultivating resilience and staying mentally flexible. Also, as we age, we need sources of strength that help us persevere, like stable romantic relationships, stable friends and support networks, religion and religious communities, and habits that keep us physically active.[336]

lyrics. However, we're in luck because now there's a translation of the lyrics into English, via Genius (Genius is the world's biggest collection of song lyrics and musical knowledge):

> Here comes a lion, father
> Oh yes it's a lion
> Here comes a lion, father
> Oh yes it's a lion
> A lion
> We're going to conquer
> A lion
> A lion and a leopard come to this open place.[214]

Lions and lionesses, ramp up your sense of hope. Sharpen your senses and your bodies. Enjoy the rest of your lives.

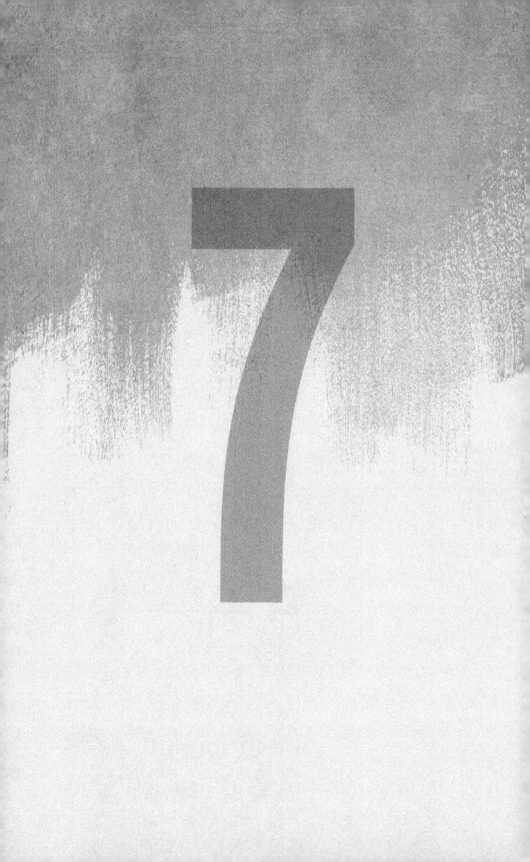

Optimal Wellness—Your Wellness Journey after Your First Hormone Replacement

In my research for *Restore* and the age-old legends of the search for the wisdom to age youthfully, I stumbled upon an old text regarding the worldwide legend of a fountain of youth. Here is a passage from this charming sixty-eight-page article published in 1905 by Dr. E. Washburn Hopkins, a Yale University professor, that explores the origins of these legends worldwide throughout history. Dr. Hopkins (1857–1932) was a Yale professor, an American Sanskrit scholar, and editor of the *Journal of the American Oriental Society*.[215]

"To find this Fountain of Youth on European soil," Dr. Hopkins observed, "we must first turn to the writers of romance, who took the myth from the East."[216]

He continues:

> In the fifteenth century, in the story of Huon de Bordeaux,
> we read that the hero discovers near the Persian Gulf the
> Fountain of Youth, which comes out of Paradise. No sooner
> has Huon bathed in this fountain than he feels resusci-
> tated from the effects of his late labours and recovers his
> pristine vigour, without the meretricious aid of magical
> drugs or enchantments. Near the fountain "grew a tree, of
> which the apples partook of the resuscitating properties
> of the water by which its roots were nourished."[217]

So our late Middle Ages hero rejuvenated himself with the fountain, and then left with apples, which had the same renewing effect.

Having some fun with this legend, I compare that with Huon drinking from the fountain. The apples he carries away represent what comes next, a wonderful metaphor for the fruits of that new wellness once your hormones have been restored. We call that optimal health. And there are many varieties of that apple.

We will be watching these results with you. All that leads to one thing, the event we're playing for, the event of life, right? So now we offer to teach you how to eat, how to exercise, how to sleep, all those things.

We'll cover diets, fasting, nutrient deficiencies, and sleep. We'll address the importance of building muscle as we age, exercise, supplement with vitamins D3 and K, and update you on the latest research and clinical effect of cholesterol, statins, progesterone, thyroid care, iodine, and peptides.

My board certifications as an MD include being board certified by the American Board of Anti-Aging and Regenerative Medicine. The aging process can be a youthful experience. We follow the latest knowledge and clinical studies and suggest ways to get your body into optimal shape for the fantastic rest of your life.

In my practice, we give our patients choices, offer them education and insight into their cellular, metabolic, and hormone health, and empower them to take control of their health.

We have found that, especially after the impact of BHRT, folks want to keep progressing. We study follow-up labs, which guide our recommendations for the next steps.

So in summary, the journey ahead can benefit from expertise for optimal hormones, sleep, nutrition, self-care, movement, metabolism, and detoxification.

We're restoring the homeostasis balance of our body. That's all we're doing. The body itself is brilliant enough to do its work. We're restoring the fuel source.

We're restoring the homeostasis balance of our body. That's all we're doing. The body itself is brilliant enough to do its work. We're restoring the fuel source. We focus on restoring your hormones, sleep, when and what you eat, exercise and muscle development, and removing stress and toxins, and we know Rome cannot be built in a day. Do it gradually, at your own pace.

Use your medical freedom. Watch the results.

Even if we never meet, I urge you to limit your eating to a five-to-eight-hour window every day (intermittent fasting). Get rid of grains and refined sugar. Eat fat and protein, and take vitamin D with K2MK-7 supplements, which will improve your life significantly. Our goal is to educate. We do need these supplements mainly because of our environment. The topsoil has been destroyed for a hundred years because of how we grow things.

So clinically, if you look at your chart, you will see notes about your thyroid, mitochondria, redox equations, AMPK, vitamin D, peptides, fasting, sleep practices, and lipogenesis, all that becomes background music as we show you the science and how all this works in the human body. You now have the fuel to succeed. You're sleeping well again and walking every day. So maybe learn a little more at your own pace. We know that handing you a list of a dozen changes to make would overwhelm you. I will suggest your next steps, and it's very OK if they are baby steps.

In his book, *Outlive: The Science and Art of Longevity*, Dr. Peter Attia describes an enzyme called AMP-activated protein kinase, or AMPK, as like the low fuel light on the dashboard of your car: when it senses low levels of nutrients (fuel), it activates, triggering a cascade of actions.

While this typically happens as a response to a lack of nutrients, "AMPK is also activated when we exercise, responding to the transient drop in nutrient levels. Just as you would change your itinerary if your fuel light came on, heading for the nearest gas station rather than Grandma's house, AMPK prompts the cell to conserve and seek alternative sources of energy."[218]

It does this, Dr. Attia explains:

> First by stimulating the production of new mitochondria, the tiny organelles that produce energy in the cell, via a process called mitochondrial biogenesis. Over time, or with disuse—our mitochondria become vulnerable to oxidative stress and genomic damage, leading to dysfunction and failure. Restricting the amount of nutrients that are available, via dietary restriction or exercise, triggers the production of new, more efficient mitochondria to replace old and damaged ones.[219]

BHRT ultimately begins to optimize hormone utilization in the body by increasing hormone sensitivity and communication at a cellular level through diet supplements and lifestyle.

230

Overall, we are supporting mitochondria and metabolic health so that hormones can work more efficiently and improve long-term health outcomes further.

> Optimal Follow-Up Intervals after BHRT:
>
> Men: Four to Six Months after BHRT
>
> Women: Three to Four Months after BHRT

We already have baseline results just prior to your pellet insertion, which guides the formulation we select for you, and possibly some supplements, such as vitamin D3 plus K and Meta 13C. After several months have passed and your body assimilates the new surge of energy, we will ask you for a follow-up blood test, another hormone panel. When your lab sends us the results, we begin to plan where to go next.

After four months, one recent male patient in his seventies reported some welcome results. His testosterone score rose from the mid-200s to 1,100. His sleep optimization, as measured by his new Oura ring, stayed in the high 90s as optimal. His average resting heart rate dropped from 67 to 54. He dropped twenty pounds in three months. His impressed pulmonary specialist tested his lung function and offered to take him off his asthma medication. His average HRV balance has been optimal every week, rising from 19 to 40, measuring how well you recover from stress, and his daily readiness score, an Oura overall score that you receive when you wake up each morning, stays in the high 90s. And his mood and mental stamina improved. I like getting this kind of data back from my patients.

HERE'S WHAT WE EXAMINE AFTER YOUR FIRST BHRT

Follow-Up Results

Priority results examined before a second placement of bioidentical hormone replacement therapy

Men

- Testosterone
- Thyroid
- Vitamin D
- PSA

Women

- (depending on age)
- Testosterone
- Estrogen (and FSH)
- Progesterone
- Thyroid
- FSH (for women who are menopausal or in the perimenopausal range)

At the close of the third or fourth month following BHRT (depending on your health factors, age, and sex), the minute our follow-up blood results arrive, our trending tells us where to go from here. We have priorities.

So the only major difference between men and women is the estrogen components. We focus on keeping the engine running. Some of the most important indicators in this bloodwork are your thyroid results. That's what we study.

What do you first think about if your car stops? For me, that's the fuel. We're driving along, and you have to coast to the side of the road. You're not going to think of an alternator. You're not going to think of an electrical disorder. You're going to think all that after you check the fuel. The sex hormones estrogen, testosterone, and progesterone are the gasoline. And for the carburetor, oxygen is the thyroid. And like a car with a broken fuel gauge, if you don't keep track of how much gas you put in, you'll never know when or where you may have to pull over to the side of the road.

After BHRT, or anytime to help you overcome a health challenge, our practice provides a structured wellness program with comprehensive counseling available. Our team can go in depth with you on how and what you eat, where you think you're healthy, and where you're not, and coach you about fasting. We make this as affordable as possible and as simple as possible. We tailor this program for BHRT patients fighting obesity, thyroid problems, or other chronic issues.

Testosterone

Think of this hormone as the lowest-hanging apple on the tree.

If your last few months have been restoring your hormones to optimal levels, you have probably seen many or most of the nefarious effects of your previous deficiency dissipate.

By the time you return to our office, testosterone deficiency has been remedied. BHRT improves well-being, strength, body composition, libido or erection, cardiovascular stability, cognitive function, mood, irritability, depression, and you have reduced your chances of osteoporosis, cardiovascular dysfunction, heart attack, stroke, and all forms of dementia.

The University of Rochester Medical Center's Health Encyclopedia reminds us of the vital importance of this hormone for both women and men.[220]

After BHRT, most of the symptoms of low T will disappear.

Symptoms of low testosterone in males include:

- Large breasts
- Low sex drive or lack of interest in sex
- Trouble getting an erection
- Low sperm count and other fertility problems
- Changes in the testicles
- Weak bones
- Irritability
- Trouble concentrating
- Loss of muscle mass
- Hair loss
- Depression
- Fatigue
- Anemia

Symptoms of low testosterone in females include:

- Fertility problems
- Missed or irregular menstrual periods
- Osteoporosis
- Low sex drive
- Changes in breast tissue
- Vaginal dryness

We also check other hormone levels, such as luteinizing hormone (LH), thyroid-stimulating hormone (TSH) and prolactin, but our priority is first to ensure that we maintain optimal restoration of the fuel for the body, testosterone.

As mentioned in our story many times, reference values vary from laboratory to laboratory. And they change all the time, seemingly at random, reacting to the basically unhealthy population.

The Mayo Clinic's 2023 published reference values for testosterone are 300–950 ng/dl (nanograms per deciliter) for young adult men and 12–60 ng/dl for young adult women.[221]

We stretch these reference values even higher to try to achieve an optimal level, based on our experience at Optimal Bio. We do not even like to hear the term "normal range."

Optimal Bio Ranges (ranges, not "limits")

- Males: 900–1,300 ng/dl
- Females: 70–250 ng/dl
- Other 2023 published reference intervals:

Labcorp[222]

- Males: 264–916 ng/dl (ages 31–80)
- (Interestingly, on June 30, 2017, this was 348 ng/dl–1,197ng/dl)
- Females: 8–60 ng/dl (ages 31–40)
- 2–45 ng/dl (over 80)

Quest Diagnostics[223]

- Males: 250–1,100 ng/dl
- Females: 2–45 ng/dl

BioReference Laboratories[224]

- Males over age 50: 193–740 ng/dl
- Males aged 19–49: 249–836 ng/dl
- Females aged 19–49: 8.4–48.1 ng/dl
- Females age 50+: 2.9–40.8 ng/dl

NEW DEVELOPMENTS IN CARING FOR
TRAUMATIC BRAIN INJURY (TBI)

Traumatic brain injury (TBI) incurs substantial health and economic burden, a leading reason for death and disability globally. Fall from height and motor vehicle crashes are the two most common causes of TBI, the latter generally affecting the economically productive population. And as we all know, thousands of American heroes suffer from lingering disabilities from TBI.

A study published by the Neuro Critical Care Society alerts the medical world to the growing evidence supporting the long-held belief that brain injuries precipitate hormone deficiency and great relief can be gained by first recognizing the often-hidden symptoms which can be mistaken for symptoms from the brain injury itself.[225] And secondly, evaluating patients through this clinical lens with an eye on hormone replacement, which offers great promise in a wide range of studies.

"Acute brain injury not only causes direct brain injury but also affects distant organs," the authors report, and the "extent of extracerebral involvement depends on the severity of the injury," the report added.[226]

Some of those distant organs could be hormone deficient as a consequence of the brain injury.

Endocrine abnormalities are no longer considered a rare complication of TBI.

236

Years ago, I wrote a white paper entitled "A Better and Safer Way to Treat PTSD." It holds true today.

PTSD is not limited to the military population. In fact, it is estimated that 5.2 million people in the US are currently suffering *from* this debilitating condition.

The brain controls the production of hormones, and many of the symptoms of PTSD are amplified by low testosterone. Chronic anxiety and depression have been proven to lower natural hormone levels, and low levels of hormones can trigger more anxiety and depression. These two conditions, sadly, worsen over time in a negative feedback loop.

So rather than masking the problem with drugs, some PTSD patients have discovered something that works better than antidepressants, specifically, bioidentical hormone replacement therapy, which is infinitely safer, in addition to being more effective.

Barrett Johnson Urges Combat Veterans with PTSD, TBI to Discover BHRT and Greatness in the Help Now Available

Barrett Johnson

Barrett Johnson began his military training at Virginia Military Institute and went directly into the Navy SEAL program from college. He served in elite and highly classified missions for a total of twenty-two years, starting at SEAL Team Two, then SEAL Team Six, then a tour at JSOC at Fort Bragg, and then SEAL Team Ten. Most of his service was in combat roles or training for missions.

Barrett says he has not been willing to talk much about his experiences. Still, his recovery has been so dramatic and powerful that he feels like his experience should be shared with every warrior recovering from the visible and invisible damage from continuous combat:

I was a breacher for fourteen years in SEAL teams. Breachers use explosives to break into a location known to be occupied by enemy combatants. So the toll that those repeated explosions take on the brain and other parts of the body is phenomenal, in a not-good way. And we didn't know any of that until fairly recently.

In 2005, I had a terrible panic attack and didn't know what was happening. This lasted for years. I could not find my way out, constantly in moderate to extreme panic. This was devastating, to the point that I was becoming hopeless. I was going to take my life. I leaned into too much alcohol to self-medicate. I was on a terrible downward spiral, just deteriorating. I could not shake it off and figure out what was wrong. I couldn't pinpoint it. It wasn't necessarily PTSD or anything like that. I certainly have that to an extent, but PTSD has never been debilitating for me. It's just kind of a thing in the background. I couldn't figure out what was going on.

And at that time from 2005 to 2008, nobody talked about that kind of stuff in the SEAL teams. I didn't have anybody I knew who had those problems I was going through. I kept it all to myself. We all did. We didn't want the stigma that might get us kicked out. I worried that guys would shun me or lose confidence in my abilities in a critical moment, so I kept it to myself, self-medicated, and contemplated suicide. I wanted to "check out of the net."

And at that point, I finally presented myself to our command psych; I didn't care if they took my clearance away. My life and my family were clearly on the line. I did that, and they were helpful. I didn't get in any trouble for it. They tried to treat me for depression with few results. I dealt with that from 2008 until 2015, a year after I retired, when the downward spiral started again, even worse.

Then on a particularly bad night, I called a friend of mine, still on active duty, a highly respected command master chief. And I just said, I'm going to end it.

And he started immediately setting the wheels in motion. Quickly, the Navy SEAL Foundation sent me to Dallas to the Cerebrum Health Center Veteran Treatment Program, where hundreds of wounded veterans have been treated for traumatic brain injury. That was a huge game changer because that was my first introduction to testosterone therapy. At that time, when I was first tested, my testosterone level was 57. And they couldn't figure out how I was even functioning.

They did a whole litany of tests and treatments over a structured two-week program, one-on-one with the doctors. This opened my eyes to many things; there is more to this than what I'd been treated for (depression or whatever else.) It was working, and it made a huge difference.

They were treating me with injectable testosterone. But the problem with that program was they would treat you for six months, and then you're supposed to transition to your primary care physician to take over that treatment. So when I transitioned, my doctor took me off everything, and I went right back to where I was, and I was very frustrated. My wife, Anna, was up in arms about that. She was soon to step in. Anna has been my best advocate even when I wouldn't advocate for myself.

One evening, not too long after that, Dr. Greg Brannon was invited by the Special Forces Association to give a speech at our local VFW, where my wife and I belong. She attended Dr. Brannon's presentation and brought all that home, saying, "You've got to see this guy. I will set you up with all the appointments and tests to see Dr. Greg Brannon. Now."

So I did.

Dr. Brannon's BHRT pellets changed everything. It leveled me out. I operate intensely, and my body responds perfectly to a testosterone level of about 1,300. That's where I try to stay with the bioidentical pellet therapy. The libido and physical aspects of it are a benefit, a nice side effect. But really, it's the mental aspect that changed my life.

BHRT took away my panic attacks for the most part. It took away the brain fog. It changed my whole mental thinking from this downward spiral to, this will be all right now. Things are great. It's such a game changer. It's almost like somebody turns the lights on like you get a sudden breath of oxygen. The first couple of times you have pellets placed, it's like, oh my God, the world's colors are brighter. I had been struggling with some pretty bad memory loss for years. BHRT helped with that immensely. I still have it, but not to the same magnitude.

This affected me: a healthier body, mind, and soul.

I look forward to seeing Dr. Brannon every four months now; It's quick and easy. You're in and out. I'm the strongest I've ever been, which is crazy. I'm fifty-two years old, but I easily bench-pressed 325 pounds last week. I have been receiving pellets for about four years now.

I still have work to do, however. I have a recent diagnosis of pseudobulbar affect (PBA), a neurological condition involving involuntary, sudden, and frequent episodes of laughing or crying, most commonly found in patients with traumatic brain injury (TBI).

The part of my brain that is still affected by the blasts is the part of my brain that controls my emotions. I was still experiencing feelings that were the exact opposite of what should have been happening. I had been trying to stuff those reverse emotions so hard, and that inflamed the panic attacks.

Now I've got a handle on it. It's not entirely gone, but it's 90 percent better. I have learned that this is rare. That may explain why I had to find out about this myself. The neuroscientists that I have seen in the past never mentioned it to me. I came across an article a couple of years ago that sounded exactly like what I am continuing to experience. This disorder seems to go through cycles. Sometimes I'm on top of the world, and then here comes a little bit of a dip. There is still uncertainty about my future as regards treatment.

I am not the kind of guy that likes talking about my health. But I see many warriors I know struggling with this same stuff, so if my story's out there, I know it can help shed some light on all this. I talk to a lot of them regularly. That was not the case for a while when I was going through my dark times. But now, I stay up with the soldiers that I feel could benefit from some advice or help from me because of what I went through. And I especially want to broadcast the PBA experience. I'm the only one I know who has had PBA, or at least knows that they have PBA, and I believe I cannot be the only one.

I offer one piece of advice to every veteran reading this and every family member of a veteran: you have to stay on top of your health passionately. You have toughed out adversity for your entire life, and you may think you're OK enough to tough it out, and that's not the correct answer. Better answers are available now. There's BHRT available for guys and gals. Get tested. Stay on top of it.

There's greatness in the help that's available, so do it.

—Barrett Johnson

ESTROGEN

The Four Types of Estrogen

E1 Estrone

E1 Estrone is the primary form of estrogen that your body makes after menopause, synthesized in the adipose tissues and adrenal glands. Can be metabolized into estradiol. When high, it increases the risk of breast cancer. Selectively binds to ERa 5:1 (proliferative). Sugar and carbohydrates in our diet cause this to become more dominant than Estradiol, which increases obesity.

E2 Estradiol

E2 Estradiol is the primary type during your reproductive years and the most potent—the product of estrogen biosynthesis. It comes from the granulose cells of the ovaries. Equally activates ERa and ERb 1:1. E2 vasodilates, increasing the blood flow to the brain, bone, skin, and sex organs. Our goal for estradiol in male patients is 25–60 pg/mL. (Excess testosterone naturally converts to E2 estradiol.)

- Increases HDL, decreases LDL, and total cholesterol

- Decreases triglycerides

- Helps maintain bone structure, increases serotonin, decreases fatigue, works as an antioxidant

- Helps maintain memory, and helps the absorption of calcium, magnesium, and zinc

- Is protective of breast tissue in young women before menopause because of the presence of estradiol

E3 Estriol

E3 Estriol is the primary type during pregnancy (increases one-thousand-fold). The adrenal glands make DHEAS, liver converts it into 16a-hydroxy-DHEAS, travels to the placenta, which converts it to E3.

- Barely detectable in absence of pregnancy, helps maintain a pregnancy

- Protective/preventative for cancers (cancer risk low in pregnancy because of E3 dominance)

- Agonist of ERa and ERb; does not have the effect on the heart, bone, and brain as estradiol does

- Helps the GI tract maintain lactobacillus, part of the triple marker prenatal testing

- Prefers to bind to beta in 3:1 ratio, used in BHRT; Protective in breast cancer, helps reduce bacteria and restore pH balance

E4 Estetrol

E4 Estetrol is a human natural estrogen that was discovered in 1965 in the urine of pregnant women. It is made by human fetal livers—moderate affinity for both ERa and ERb, with a preference for ERa. Clinical studies have demonstrated possible use as estrogen in combined oral contraceptives (COC).

The Role of Estrogen in Women and Men

ESTROGEN LEVELS

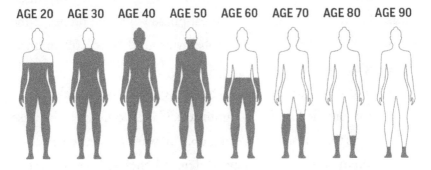

The Pulse, Estrogen Deficiency: Before, During, and After pregnancy, https://blog.pregistry.com/estrogen-deficiency-pregnancy/, accessed January 22, 2023.

Estrogen deficiency: Before, during, and after pregnancy

When a woman enters her reproductive age, her estrogen and FSH change daily, every single day, until ovulation, and then it still changes daily, and progesterone is zero. It will look very low until ovulation, peaks around 10 and goes back down. It drops after ovulation on day 14, then goes back down to the next cycle, then progesterone goes up to about 10, and on day 21 it goes down.

When women experience their period, their FSH is around 8 to 10. And then, as the ovary makes testosterone which converts to estrogen, the higher the estradiol goes, the lower the estrogen is. When estradiol hits around 200 to 400 picograms per deciliter, then the SSH in the gonadotropin is changed to LH, and that makes the egg release the progesterone from the corpus luteum, and then the estrogen drops.

When I give supplemental estrogen, the FSH (follicle-stimulating hormone) will drop as it's exposed to the estrogen. The brain thinks the ovaries are now making more eggs again, it isn't, but hormonally it is.

So, in a cycling woman, every day can be a different number. That's why knowing why you're doing it is very important. If I am working to solve infertility, I always try to get blood drawn on day 21 because days 21 to 24 are the optimal days for a woman's progesterone. I'm trying to mimic the luteal phase when the progesterone is around 5 to 10, the estrogen probably around 50 to 100, and the FCH under 10.

I am looking at trending on that more than anything else.

A protein called BCL-2 is significant. Cancer cells love it because that protects them from being eaten up. You want to have low BCL-2. And different receptor sites have different benefits. Like progesterone, a receptor increases BCL-2. Progesterone B receptors decrease it. Membrane receptors increase it; genomic decreases it.

PROGESTERONE

Progesterone, a cholesterol derivative, has numerous important functions in the human body. In males, progesterone functions to facilitate spermiogenesis and androgen synthesis. Progesterone is a precursor to testosterone, produced by the Leydig cells in the testes.

It has recently been studied for its protective role in neurological disorders. Progesterone has been shown to regulate cognition, reduce inflammation, improve mitochondrial function, stimulate neurogenesis and myelination, and help recover from traumatic brain injuries.

It is primarily associated with regulating the female reproductive system and more. It also plays a large part in reducing cancer risk, stimulating bone formation, optimizing thyroid function and testosterone synthesis, and repair of the central and peripheral nervous systems.

Progesterone helps synthesize other hormones, has many neuroprotective properties, reduces ovarian, endometrial, and breast cancer, helps to alleviate brain fog, insomnia, anxiety, depression, abnormal uterine bleeding, reduces symptoms of PCOS and endometriosis, and reduces miscarriage and infertility.

Progesterone stimulates the production of thyroid peroxidase (TPO) which synthesizes thyroxine (T4) and triiodothyronine (T3). Progesterone treatment in women with hypothyroidism works to significantly lower TSH and a significant increase in free T4.

Patients of premenopausal age are still making adequate estrogen, but as they become closer to menopause, decreasing progesterone synthesis takes place, causing estrogen dominance. These patients can present with normal estrogen, TSH, T3, and T4; however, they exhibit symptoms of fatigue, weight gain, constipation, temperature dysregulation, brain fog, depression, muscle aches, and weakness all attributed to low progesterone levels.[227]

Progesterone and synthetic progestins are not remotely the same. Understanding the actions of the progesterone receptors helps understand the different actions that occur in response to bioidentical progesterone versus synthetic progestins. Progesterone is protective, while synthetic progestins are carcinogenic.[228]

Synthroid (synthetic) versus Armour Thyroid (bioidentical)

Armour Thyroid

- Bioidentical thyroid hormones (T3 and T4)

- Must be taken either one hour prior to eating or two hours after eating

- Best if given twice daily (once in a.m. and once in p.m.) due to the half-life of T3 being about seven hours

Synthroid (Levothyroxine)

Synthetic T4

- Most commonly used thyroid treatment in the United States.

- If a patient is a poor converter of T4 to T3, they likely will convert a majority of the T4 to RT3.

- Occasionally patients will be ideally treated with Synthroid and do not want to switch treatments. Those patients should continue care for thyroid with their prescriber.

- Progesterone deficiency can lead to:

  - increased risk for endometrial, breast, and ovarian cancers

  - fatigue

  - weight gain

  - decreased bone density

  - brain fog

  - depression

  - anxiety

  - abnormal uterine bleeding

  - PCOS (polycystic ovary syndrome)

  - endometriosis

  - miscarriage

  - infertility

- amenorrhea (absence of a menstrual period)

- hair loss

- insomnia

- low libido

- hot flashes

- breast tenderness

- low blood sugar[229]

Natural progesterone protects against breast cancer, decreases fluid retention, makes normal glucose, lowers LDL and cholesterol, and protects against anxiety. Synthetic progestin counteracts the protection of estradiol, but natural progesterone enhances it.

OUR TOXIC ENVIRONMENT

The most common environmental cause of low progesterone is exposure and inability to metabolize endocrine-disrupting compounds (EDCs), synthetic chemical products used as industrial solvents, and lubricants. This also includes their byproducts: polychlorinated biphenyls (PCBs), polybrominated biphenyls (PBBs), dioxins, plastics like bisphenol A (BPA), plasticizers (phthalates), pesticides methoxychlor, chlorpyrifos, dichlorodiphenyltrichloroethane (DDT), fungicides, as well as pharmaceutical agents diethylstilbestrol (DES).[230]

There seems to be an association between exposure to these chemicals early in development (fetus or young child) and significant disease processes later in life. EDCs disrupt hormone synthesis by binding to receptor sites throughout the body. This binding causes an artificial stimulation of the negative feedback loop and thus further lowering of hormone levels. EDCs have been linked to low hormones, numerous carcinomas, male hypogonadism, male and female infertility, PCOS, male and female reproductive tract abnormalities, uterine leiomyomas, endometriosis, and neural disease.[231]

We always do oral progesterone. If your progesterone is low, we see that patients experience anxiety, increased depression, increased breast tenderness, bloatedness, fluid retention, mood swings, and messed up sleep. We'll check your level, and if you need a supplement, we will do it orally. We use this delivery method because in this case, oral intake converts to allopregnanolone, a protective neurosteroid, a big advantage over the cream method. It's a neurosteroid which can enhance learning and memory and exhibits anti-inflammatory effects.

Progesterone from a compounding pharmacy is derived from the plant byproduct diosgenin. This phytosteroid comes from wild yams and serves as the basic chemical structure for progesterone. Once introduced into the human body, the body cannot differentiate between progesterone produced by the compounding pharmacy or progesterone produced by the human body itself. Compounded progesterone has the same chemical and structural make-up as endogenous progesterone. Bioidentical progesterone binds harmoniously to its receptors throughout the body.

This same structural unity is not seen when synthetic progestins bind to progesterone receptors. When such synthetic chemicals enter the system, they can not only activate progesterone receptors but also attach to other cell receptors, thus eliciting unwanted side effects.

THYROID

Your thyroid creates and produces hormones that play a role in many different systems, all supervised by the pituitary gland. Located in the center of the skull, below your brain, the pituitary gland monitors and controls the amount of thyroid hormones in your bloodstream.

"The risk for women to have a thyroid disorder in their lifetime is five to eight times greater than for a man"[232]

When your thyroid makes either too much or too little of these essential hormones, it's called thyroid disease. There are several different types of thyroid disease, including hyperthyroidism, hypothyroidism, thyroiditis, and Hashimoto's thyroiditis. When the pituitary gland senses a lack of thyroid hormones or a high level of hormones in your body, it will adjust the amounts with its own hormone. This hormone is called thyroid-stimulating hormone (TSH). The TSH will be sent to the thyroid, telling the thyroid what needs to be done to get the body back to normal.

> **The risk for women to have a thyroid disorder in their lifetime is five to eight times greater than for a man.**

The Cleveland Clinic notes that the risk for women to have a thyroid disorder in their lifetime is five to eight times greater than for a man.[233] Millions of men experience thyroid dysfunction, but women are more likely to have a thyroid imbalance.

Symptoms of an overactive thyroid (hyperthyroidism) can include:

- Experiencing anxiety, irritability, and nervousness
- Having trouble sleeping
- Losing weight
- Having an enlarged thyroid gland or a goiter
- Having muscle weakness and tremors
- Experiencing irregular menstrual periods or having your menstrual cycle stop
- Feeling sensitive to heat

- Having vision problems or eye irritation[234]

Symptoms of an underactive thyroid (hypothyroidism) can include:

- Feeling tired (fatigue)

- Gaining weight

- Experiencing forgetfulness

- Having frequent and heavy menstrual periods

- Having dry and coarse hair

- Having a hoarse voice

- Experiencing an intolerance to cold temperatures[235]

In regulating the body's metabolism and growth, the thyroid gland secretes several hormones:

- Thyroxine (T4)

- Triiodothyronine (T3)

- Calcitonin

The functions of the thyroid gland have much to do with a woman's reproductive system, particularly if the thyroid is overactive or underactive. This hormone level imbalance may significantly affect a woman's body.

While some practitioners only order a blood test for thyroid stimulating hormone (TSH), as a result, millions of people suffering from thyroid dysfunction are left undiagnosed. Optimal thyroid function regulates weight, energy levels, internal temperature, skin, hair, nail growth, and metabolism, paramount in maintaining the body's homeostasis.

Thyroid Management Protocol

We begin a Thyroid Management Protocol as soon as a new patient arrives. If your initial labs are concerning (or abnormal), we suggest beginning supplements and reevaluating after six months. When we see the T3 is under 3.4, we'll suggest adding supplements first.

During the initial physical exam, we'll palpate (feel for nodules, etc.) your thyroid area.

If we decide to medicate, we'll recheck the labs in eight weeks, and if it is stable after that, we'll recheck after six months.

We keep the running results as we advance with our Thyroid Flow Sheet and Thyroid Document for every initial and follow-up visit.

Thyroid Optimal Levels

TSH 0.5-2

- Free T4 (greater than) 1.1
- Free T3 (greater than) 3.4
- RT3 (less than)10
- TPO (less than) 9
- TGA 0–0.9
- Mitochondrial antibody (less than) 20
- Ferritin 50–100

Possible Thyroid Treatments

- Supplementation Only

We suggest supplements for our patients with lab values to suggest a slightly dysfunctional thyroid. These patients could have some symptoms of hypothyroid or maybe no symptoms, but the labs are just slightly off.

We also agree to a supplement strategy with a patient whose thyroid is underfunctioning, but the patient does not want to start medication just yet. This would be an excellent route to go.

Recommended supplements:
- Iodoral
- Thyrosol
- Recheck labs in six months
- Supplementation + Prescription Medication

Our team uses Armour Thyroid most commonly. Occasionally, a patient will come to us while taking NP Thyroid, and it is OK for them to stay on that.

For patients that come to us already on Synthroid (Levothyroxine) and their lab values are less than ideal, we suggest switching from Synthroid to Armour Thyroid. We can also begin adding supplementation.

Labs would need to be repeated six to eight weeks from treatment initiation and continue that way until the patient is on a stable dose. At that point, the patient can have labs done at six months.

We test for Free T3 (FT3), Reverse T3 (RT3), and the presence of two thyroid antibodies, TPOAb and TgAb. The "Free" in front of T3 discloses what is unbound and usable by the body. Reverse T3 is the opposite of T3; it blocks thyroid receptors and can cause patients to be unresponsive to any thyroid hormone.

When studying the blood test results, when we see that your levels are decent (close but not perfect), then we pay very close attention to your continuing symptoms. We may hear about cold intolerance, belly fat, and brain fog. There are a lot of things that correlate with the thyroid and testosterone because they work together.

More about the Specific Blood Tests for Your Thyroid:

TSH

Most of the time, thyroid hormone deficiency (hypothyroidism) is associated with an elevated TSH level, while thyroid hormone excess (hyperthyroidism) is associated with a low TSH level.

If TSH is abnormal, measurement of thyroid hormones directly, including thyroxine (T4) and triiodothyronine (T3), may be done to further evaluate the problem.

Normal TSH range for an adult: 0.40–4.50 mIU/mL (milli-international units per liter of blood).

The standard ranges say anything under five is good. That's terrible. **I want it under 1.**

Free T4

Free T4 or free thyroxine is a method of measuring T4 that eliminates the effect of proteins that naturally bind T4 and may prevent accurate measurement.

Normal FT4 range for an adult: 0.9–1.7 ng/dL (nanograms per deciliter of blood)

Free T4 (not the total T4), the free T4. **I want it over 1.1.**

Free T3

Free T3 or free triiodothyronine is a method of measuring T3 that eliminates the effect of proteins that naturally bind T3 and may prevent accurate measurement. T4 is made a 4:1 ratio to T3. T4 is a prohormone. It's not active. T3 is active. Immediately, your thyroid squirts out the active one, which is 25 percent of the volume of the nonactive one.

The nonactive one, T4, converts to T3 with selenium. You have it over seven-day periods; you have more of it. But it also converts to what's called an enantiomer (or mirror image of it), called reverse T3.

Consider this: if we're in our car, the T3 is the gas, and the reverse T3 is the brakes. That ratio is more important than anything else. T3 ultimately makes the mitochondria turn oxygen into energy, oxygen into carbon dioxide, and water.

Normal FT3 range: 2.3–4.1 pg/mL (picograms per milliliter of blood)

Free T3

I look for over 3.4. If T3 is under 3.4, close to three, I'll add the supplements first. If not, I'll suggest medication.

Reverse T3 (RT3)

The hypothalamus makes a thing called thyroid-releasing hormone, which then goes to the anterior pituitary, makes the thyroid-stimulating hormone, which then goes to your neck. Picture a bow tie, right? You have a bow tie on your neck. That's the thyroid gland.

The thyroid gland uses selenium, iodine, zinc, vitamin C, vitamin B, tyrosine, and amino acid. It makes these hormones called T1, T2, T3, T4. (We do not know what T1 and T2 do. They are probably transition forms.) T4 and T3 are the hormones that our body makes.

Reverse T3, I look for under 10.

> **IODINE AND YOUR THYROID**
>
> There's an enzyme called TPO that makes this work in these irons.
>
> I want the **ferritin level between 50 and 100**. And then, I check the antibodies.

TPO

Thyroid Peroxidase Antibody

Less than 9 IU/mL

TPA

Thyroglobulin Antibody

0.0-0.9 IU/ml

Ferritin

50-100 ng/mL

Iodine is a mineral found in some foods. The body needs iodine to make thyroid hormones. These hormones control the body's metabolism and many other important functions. The body also needs thyroid hormones for proper bone and brain development during pregnancy and infancy. Getting enough iodine is important for everyone, especially infants and women who are pregnant.

Hashimoto's disease is an autoimmune hypothyroid that occurs when the body produces an antibody that attacks itself. Why does your body make an antibody to attack itself? You have your gut, which is one cell thick: picture *brick and mortar*. The mortar is held together by these proteins called zonulin and occludin. The gluten molecule is very toxic; if it breaks through that mortar, your body will attack it. The problem is that molecule that attacks the gluten, the antibody, also cross-reacts with the thyroid. And if it attacks the TPO protein or the TGA protein, that's Hashimoto's disease. If it attacks the mitochondria, that's hyperthyroid, which is called Graves' disease.

And here's the big kicker for the iodine.

In America, fifty years ago we ate about 20 milligrams of iodine daily. And if you look at the periodic table, you have halogens, chemical elements that include fluorine, chlorine, bromine, iodine, and astatine. Halogen comes from Greek terms meaning "produce sea salt."[236]

All of those elements are poisonous except for iodine, which is necessary.

How Much Iodine Do We Need?

The amount of iodine you need each day depends on your age. Average daily recommended amounts are listed below in micrograms (mcg).[237]

LIFE STAGE	RECOMMENDED AMOUNT
Birth to 6 months	110 mcg
Infants 7–12 months	130 mcg
Children 1–8 years	90 mcg
Children 9–13 years	120 mcg
Teens 14–18 years	150 mcg
Adults	150 mcg
Pregnant teens and women	220 mcg
Breastfeeding teens and women	290 mcg

The National Institutes of Health notes that iodine occurs naturally in some foods and is also added to salt that is labeled as "iodized."[238] You can get recommended amounts of iodine by eating a variety of foods, including the following:

- Fish (such as cod and tuna), seaweed, shrimp, and other seafood, which are generally rich in iodine

- Dairy products (such as milk, yogurt, and cheese) and eggs, which are also good sources of iodine

- Iodized salt, which is readily available in the United States and many other countries*

  *Processed foods, such as canned soups, almost never contain iodized salt. In addition, specialty salts, such as sea salt, kosher salt, Himalayan salt, and fleur de sel, are not usually iodized.

Product labels will indicate if the salt is "iodized" or provides iodine.[239]

They took iodine out of our food in the 1970s, and they put bromine in our salt and in our food instead. (I still don't get that.) Gulf War syndrome is bromine poisoning. Bromine is in a lot of pesticides; it's very bad. So they eventually replaced that.

Today, the average American day eats around 100 micrograms, 200 times less iodine. [240]

So now we have a much higher rate of thyroid disease. People think it's genetic. It's not genetic. It's because the environment beats everybody up. When you increase your iodine, you see antibodies go down and see disease go down. It's a spectrum, from the hyper to the hypo.

We have a sodium iodine pump that puts iodine in primary glandular cells, like the breast or prostate. And by doing that, it does something very interesting. It decreases breast cancer. Seaweed is an important dietary component and a rich source of iodine in several chemical forms in Asian communities. Their high consumption of this element (twenty-five times higher than in Western countries) has been associated with the low incidence of benign and cancerous breast and prostate disease in Japanese people.[241]

The more iodine you have, the gland gets saturated by around three milligrams, after that it does its other functions. It then makes what's called a lipoprotein called delta-iodolactone, known to scavenge and kill cancer cells.

Several tissues share with the thyroid gland the capacity to actively accumulate iodine; these include the salivary glands, gastric mucosa, lactating mammary gland, the choroid plexus, ciliary body of the eye, lacrimal gland, thymus, skin, placenta, ovary, uterus, prostate, and pancreas, and they may either maintain or lose this ability under pathological conditions.[242]

In other words, we all need to watch our iodine.

I had the honor of being on several broadcasts with Dr. David Brownstein a few years ago. Dr. Brownstein is one of the world's leading authorities on iodine and the thyroid. He is a board-certified family physician and one of the foremost practitioners of holistic medicine. He is the Medical Director of the Center for Holistic Medicine in West Bloomfield, Michigan. He has published fifteen books on holistic health. Two of his books are medical classics: one titled *Thyroid* and the other called *Iodine.*

BUSTING THE IODINE MYTHS

Presented with permission by Dr. David Brownstein

I am frequently asked by my patients: "If you only had one natural item to treat with, which would it be?" Although there are many natural items that provide wonderful effects for the body, one nutrient stands head and shoulders above the rest: iodine.

There are many myths about iodine, but I will focus on two main myths propagated by many conventional doctors.

Myth No. 1 is that we get enough iodine in salt, and Myth No. 2, that taking iodine as a supplement will cause or worsen thyroid disorders. Because of these myths, people have the mistaken idea that iodine is a toxic substance that needs to be avoided.

The iodization of salt was hailed as the first public health miracle. However, iodized salt is inadequate for supplying the body's need for iodine, particularly in our toxic environment. Even though refined salt can prevent goiter in the vast majority of people, the minuscule amount of iodine found in it falls far short of the amount necessary for promoting optimal thyroid function.

Furthermore, refined salt fails to provide enough iodine for the rest of the body's needs.

Iodine is added to table salt at 100 parts per million as potassium iodide, which amounts to 77 µg (micrograms) of iodide per gram of salt. (µg is the symbol for the metric measurement microgram which is one-millionth of a gram or one-thousandth of a milligram.)

The RDA for iodine is set at 150 µg per day for adults in the US and slightly more during pregnancy and lactation. Remember, the RDA was set to prevent goiter in the vast majority of people. The average American takes in 4–10 grams of refined salt per day. That's more than the recommended daily allowance. So, why don't we get enough iodine from salt?

Research shows that just 10 percent of iodine in salt is bioavailable—that is, completely absorbed by your body. Thus, iodized salt provides somewhere between 30–77 µg a day, which is markedly below the recommended amount. Additionally, approximately 70 percent of the salt used by commercial industry in the US is not iodized salt.[243]

Not only is iodized salt a poor source of iodine, but we have been conditioned to avoid salt by the media and by mainstream medicine. Presently, less than half of US households use salt. As a result, iodine levels have fallen by more than 50 percent over the last forty years as reported by the National Health and Nutrition Examination Survey from the Centers for Disease Control.[244] This is a recipe for making a whole population of US citizens iodine-deficient. That is exactly what has happened in the United States and many other Western countries.

If Myth No. 2 were correct, taking iodine will cause thyroid disorders and the declining iodine levels would help prevent thyroid disease. This has not been the case. As iodine levels have fallen over 50 percent during the last 40 years, thyroid disorders including hypothyroidism, Hashimoto's disease, Graves' disease, and thyroid cancer have been increasing at near-epidemic rates. We would expect the opposite to occur—thyroid illnesses on the decline—if iodine were the cause.

After twenty years of practicing medicine, I can state that it is impossible to treat thyroid illness if there is an inadequate level of iodine in the body, and this includes autoimmune thyroid disorders. The largest amounts of iodine occur in the oceans. Sea vegetables and ocean fish contain large amounts of iodine and are the foods that provide the most usable iodine for the body. Diets lacking in seafood can predispose one to iodine deficiency.

The recommended daily allowance for iodine, 150 mcg/day, is inadequate to supply the body's need for iodine. When you couple in the increasing exposure to toxic halides such as bromine, fluoride, and chlorine derivatives, our iodine requirements have markedly increased over the years. My experience has shown that iodine in doses ranging from 6–50 mg/day is adequate to provide iodine for most of the population.[245]

–Dr. David Brownstein

More information about this can be found in Dr. David Brownstein's books *Iodine: Why You Need It, Why You Can't Live Without It, 5th Edition* and Salt Your Way *To Health, 2nd Edition.*

Physicians used Armor Thyroid for years. Armour Thyroid is compounded, made from pigs. And for some reason, it's the exact same cell structure as ours. The same for T1, T2, T3, T4, a four-to-one ratio. Exactly the same. This is quite different from the synthetic female pregnant horse urine. That horse urine is not the same as our estrogen. Yet, in this case, the pig is identical. Estrogen is the one exception to my "no-farm-animals policy" because, despite the source, this estrogen is bioidentical, not synthetic.

Give what the body needs, exactly. Let's give it what it makes, not what some folks think it makes. The body needs iodine and selenium.

Gluten

Now the antibody parts—if you still have antibodies, we try to take people off gluten.

Often, we eliminate gluten, as well as grains. We give patients selenium, iodine, vitamin C, and other supplements, and we recheck levels in six months. If we ask you to go on medicines, I check your levels in two months.

Taking Iodine

Now Dr. Brownstein himself found his antibodies go down by adding iodine. I am currently up to 50 milligrams a day. And for most of my patients, I carefully build up to that point.

People who take iodine may have unpleasant side effects. Usually nausea, perhaps a headache. Why? It's the bromine being displaced by the iodine. Bromine is in the cell, being displaced by iodine before you urinate or excrete the bromine out. There is a way to protect you from that. Drink a quarter teaspoon of Himalayan salt in eight ounces of water, and that will make you pee out the bromine faster.

The Effectiveness of Low-Dose Naltrexone (LDN)

The TPO antibody. If that's above 10, that means you have Hashimoto's disease. The TGA antibody above 1 also means you have Hashimoto's.

The TPO antibody of my wife, Jody, at one time was sky-high. We prescribed selenium and iodine, changed her to Armour, and started low-dose naltrexone. Her antibodies are down to 100 now, which is significant for her.

Dr. David Brownstein and I have talked at length about low-dose naltrexone. He's a wonderful practitioner of allopathic and holistic together, a true pioneer in thyroid disease.

Dr. Brownstein does not use LDN. (That comes from my personal experience.) My compound pharmacist suggested LDN for me, and I have been a believer ever since. Dr. Brownstein has found that high-dose iodine (or optimal-dose iodine) will lower antibodies on its own. So that's our first line of defense. If that doesn't work out, we'll suggest LDN as well. The future of LDN is huge.

What is LDN? Naltrexone was born in the 1980s, and it's been in medical use at 50 to 300 milligrams ever since. Low-dose naltrexone, LDN was started in 1988. When prescribing the standard dose (25 milligrams and up), naltrexone acts primarily to block opiate receptors. And as such, it is used mainly in addiction. When it is used in low doses, it is now widely understood to act as an immune modulator. That's it, an immune modulator. Multiple phase one and two trials have demonstrated the efficiency of low-dose as a therapeutic agent. Low-dose naltrexone does not suppress the immune system.[246]

When used in lower doses, LDN is an immune modulator that has opiate blocking and antitumor effects. LDN is a useful treatment option if there's autoimmune or inflammatory disease. That's Hashimoto's disease and Graves' disease. LDN approves immune response. It increases the production of endorphins, promoting increase in the number of T lymphocytes. It acts directly on immune cells to stimulate restored normal immune functions.

LDN is tolerated in most patients. However, we take care to titrate up slowly to avoid side effects. So we start at very low doses. You start at 1mg and work your way up, slowly, to 5 mg, to avoid sleep disturbances, mild headache, nausea, flulike symptoms, and sometimes a rash or dizziness. The half-life is four to six hours.

Gluten-Free Diet

Optimal thyroid function maintains the body's homeostasis, regulating weight, energy levels, internal temperature, skin, hair, nail growth, and metabolism.

If labs reveal positive antibodies, this is suggestive of Hashimoto's.

In developing countries, the biggest contributor to hypothyroidism is iodine deficiency. In countries where iodine is added to table salt to ensure sufficient iodine intake, Hashimoto's (an autoimmune disorder in which antibodies attack the thyroid) is the most common cause of hypothyroidism. Anti-TPO antibodies, TGA, and antimitochondria (M2) antibodies are scrutinized in all patients at initial evaluation.

Patients with antimitochondrial antibody and thyroid labs that are normal or suggestive of hypothyroidism should have antibodies rechecked in six months.

A gluten-free diet is key to helping relieve symptoms. Low-dose naltrexone is another option in individuals with Hashimoto's and a significantly underfunctioning thyroid.

Patients with positive antimitochondrial antibodies and hyperthyroid labs are referred to endocrinology for care. This can be suggestive of Graves' disease in patients who have labs to suggest hyperthyroidism.

Although continued research is needed, it is possible that molecular mimicry is behind the relationship between gluten and Hashimoto's. During molecular mimicry, the body produces antibodies to a component that is similar in peptide structure yet still molecularly different than the structure the body is programmed to attack. The peptide structure, or physical shape, of gluten and thyroid tissue is similar, which could stimulate a cross-activation autoimmune response.

Think of a key that is close enough in shape to another key that it can unlock a door it wasn't intended to open. For example, when a person with Hashimoto's consumes gluten, the body could mistake that gluten for the thyroid, stimulating an attack on the thyroid. Naltrexone in small doses can be helpful in Hashimoto's disease. At low doses, naltrexone is a modulator of the immune system.

The same is true of a person with celiac disease—although that person may follow a gluten-free diet, the body could mistake the thyroid tissue for gluten and mount an attack on the thyroid.

Vitamin D

Vitamin D (also referred to as "calciferol") is a fat-soluble vitamin that is naturally present in a few foods, added to others, and available as a dietary supplement. It is also produced endogenously when ultraviolet (UVB) rays from sunlight strike the skin and trigger vitamin D synthesis.

Vitamin D obtained from sun exposure, foods, and supplements is biologically inert and must undergo two hydroxylations in the body for activation. The first hydroxylation, which occurs in the liver, converts vitamin D to 25-hydroxyvitamin D (25(OH)D), also known as "calcidiol." The second hydroxylation occurs primarily in the kidney and forms the physiologically active 1,25-dihydroxyvitamin D (1,25(OH)2D), also known as "calcitriol"[247]

This vitamin promotes calcium absorption in the gut and maintains adequate serum calcium and phosphate concentrations to enable normal bone mineralization and to prevent hypocalcemic tetany (involuntary contraction of muscles, leading to cramps and spasms). It is also needed for bone growth and bone remodeling by osteoblasts and osteoclasts. Without sufficient vitamin D, bones can become thin, brittle, or misshapen. Vitamin D sufficiency prevents rickets in children and osteomalacia in adults. Together with calcium, vitamin D also helps protect older adults from osteoporosis.

VITAMIN D DEFICIENCY
Affects Every Part of the Body

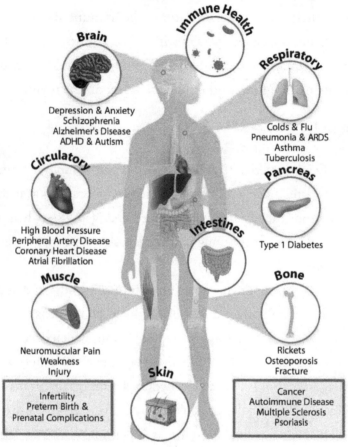

Grassroots Health Image, Vitamin D Deficiency Affects Every Part of the Body, https://www.grassrootshealth.net/document/interactive-pdf-vitamin-d-deficiency-affects-every-part-body/, accessed August 19, 2023.

Dr. Joseph Mercola, a board-certified family medicine osteopathic physician (DO), *New York Times* best-selling author and Fellow of the American College of Nutrition, estimates that up to 85 percent of people have insufficient levels of vitamin D and are unaware of their deficient state. While conventional media and medicine promote sun avoidance, "doing so can actually put your health in grave danger and cause vitamin D deficiency."[248]

A growing body of evidence shows that vitamin D plays a crucial role in disease prevention and maintaining optimal health. There are about thirty thousand genes in your body, and vitamin D affects nearly three thousand of them, as well as vitamin D receptors located throughout your body. In the largest-ever randomized clinical trial testing vitamin D for cancer prevention, the supplement did not reduce the risk of developing cancer.[249]

"A large body of epidemiology research had suggested that people with higher blood levels of vitamin D have a lower risk of cancer,"[250] said Barry Kramer, MD, director of NCI's Division of Cancer Prevention.

However, such studies can only highlight associations, not prove cause and effect, he added. "This is why it's important to question intuitions and observational epidemiology studies, and fund large-scale trials," Dr. Kramer continued; they can conclusively show whether a treatment—in this case, a dietary supplement—truly can help to prevent cancer.[251]

The VITAL trial "was well designed," said Dr. Kramer. "And when it's important to get the answer right—that is, when you're potentially making recommendations to hundreds of thousands, or even millions, you want to make sure that your recommendations are based on very strong evidence," he added.[252]

Other research into vitamin D and cancer prevention is ongoing, such as studying whether some types of cancer may be more sensitive than others to the effects of supplementation.

Results from the trial called the Vitamin D and Omega-3 Trial (VITAL), were published November 10, 2018, in the *New England Journal of Medicine* (*NEJM*).

We believe Vitamin D can help reduce the risk of other conditions as well, including type 2 diabetes, chronic inflammation, age-related macular degeneration (the leading cause of blindness), and Alzheimer's disease. Vitamin D also exhibits its infection-fighting abilities in the treatment of tuberculosis, pneumonia, colds, and flu. It can also improve seizure control in epileptics.

While scientists refer to vitamin D as a vitamin, it is actually a steroid hormone obtained from sun exposure, food sources, and supplementation. Common types of vitamin D are vitamin D2 and D3. Compared to D2, vitamin D3 is 87 percent more effective, and is the preferred form for addressing insufficient levels of vitamin D.

Today, many Americans are found to be in a serious deficiency state. A large percentage of senior citizens in the United States may possibly be deficient, far below optimal levels.[253]

Another critical point to remember is you shouldn't take any vitamin D supplement without taking vitamin K2. Vitamin K2 deficiency is connected to vitamin D toxicity symptoms, which includes excessive calcification that can contribute to the hardening of your arteries. Dr. Mercola recommends a level of 60 to 80 ng/mL.

One of the functions of vitamin K2 is to direct calcium to areas in your body where it is needed, such as your bones and teeth. It also functions to keep calcium away from areas where it shouldn't be, including your soft tissues and arteries.

According to Dr. Kate Rheaume-Bleue, author of *Vitamin K2 and the Calcium Paradox: How a Little-Known Vitamin Could Save Your Life*, When you take vitamin D, she states:

> Your body creates more of these vitamin K2-dependent proteins, the proteins that will move the calcium around. They have a lot of potential health benefits. But until the K2 comes in to activate those proteins, those benefits

aren't realized. So, really, if you're taking vitamin D, you're creating an increased demand for K2. And vitamin D and K2 work together to strengthen your bones and improve your heart health.[254]

For so long, Dr. Rheaume-Bleue says:

We've been told to take calcium for osteoporosis ... and vitamin D, which we know is helpful. But then, more studies are coming out showing that increased calcium intake is causing more heart attacks and strokes. That created a lot of confusion around whether calcium is safe or not. But that's the wrong question to be asking because we'll never properly understand the health benefits of calcium or vitamin D unless we take into consideration K2. That's what keeps the calcium in its right place.[255]

I recommend supplementing with 5,000–10,000 IU with K2-MK7 per day, depending on your lab levels. It is important to take your vitamin D with a meal that contains some fat with a high-quality vitamin K supplement for the best absorption.

Dr. Mercola notes that there is much more to vitamin D than meets the eye. Excessive vitamin D could result in overcalcification, so the body makes vitamin D in the skin upon exposure to solar ultra-violet radiation, stores it in the liver, keeping a few months' supply to get through winter, then converts it to its active form (calcitriol). Vitamin D in the blood is predominantly the bound form, with about 1 percent being unbound and bioavailable.

The crux of vitamin D metabolism is that it must be metabolized in the kidneys to its active form, calcitriol.

What is the bottom-line delivery of vitamin D to our body?

The human body limits the amount of vitamin D available to prevent overcalcification, vitamin D being the regulator of calcium availability. So vitamin D3 is synthesized in the skin, shuttled to the liver for storage (as calcidiol), and released on an as-needed basis, being transported via the vitamin D binding protein to the kidneys, where it is enzymatically metabolized into the active form of vitamin D (calcitriol).

Around 85 to 90 percent of vitamin D (calcidiol) released from the liver is bound to the vitamin D binding protein, and 10-15 percent is bound to albumin, so less than 1 percent is the active unbound (free) vitamin D (calcitriol).

The disconnect is that customarily blood laboratories only measure how much unmetabolized vitamin D3 is in circulation in the bloodstream, not how much active vitamin D (calcitriol) is available. Advances in testing now make it possible to measure activated (free, unbound) vitamin D.

Dr. Mercola notes that you can't possibly overdose on sunshine vitamin D. He suggests:

- Supplementing with 8,000 IU of vitamin D per day

- Supplementing your diet with zinc and selenium to activate vitamin D[256]

There is more to this vitamin D story every day. New developments in vitamin D metabolism are underway. Stand by.

In 2023, the *International Journal of Environmental Research and Public Health* published a study that observed that relatively consistent evidence exists for an inverse association between vitamin D status and all-cause mortality.[257]

Vitamin D plays a role in avoiding numerous diseases, including:

- Cancer

- Diabetes

- Acute respiratory tract infections

- Chronic inflammatory diseases

- Autoimmune diseases such as multiple sclerosis

It's important to note that vitamin D supplementation must be balanced with other nutrients, namely vitamin K2 (to avoid complications associated with excessive calcification in your arteries), calcium, and magnesium. Your results will indicate whether we should recommend another insertion of pellets as a booster and what supplements we should consider in the coming months. This is hopefully a face-to-face discussion. We can examine your record, your weight, discuss your now-youthful blood chemistry results, and see where you want to go next.

PSA Test

We always include the PSA test for male patients in our bloodwork for BHRT. I am not fond of the science behind this test. Over the past fifteen years, public health authorities have downgraded recommendations for the prostate-specific antigen (PSA) test as a screening tool to reduce the overdiagnosis and overtreatment of men with low-grade prostate cancer.

I always have a conversation with every male patient about the controversy and the science behind the test. Here are the facts. Make your own decision.

Although "no appropriately designed and powered study has been conducted to assess prostate cancer-related risks of testosterone therapy (TT), the available evidence suggests that TT does not increase prostate cancer risk."[258]

Actually, men with *low levels* of testosterone are associated with higher rates of prostate cancer as well as more advanced prostate cancer tumor grade, stage, and volume compared with men who are not hypogonadal.[259]

"Observational studies also suggest that men taking testosterone do not have an increased risk of developing prostate cancer. A large longitudinal study evaluating roughly 10,000 men found no association between androgen levels and prostate cancer risk," the study concluded.[260]

According to the American Cancer Society, about one in eight men will be diagnosed with the disease in their lifetime.[261] But the cancer is often slow-growing and may never progress to the point of threatening a man's life: about one in every forty-one men die of the disease.[262]

That's why routine screening, with blood tests that measure a protein called PSA, has been controversial. The main concern is that it may often detect small tumors that would never have become harmful, leading to "overtreatment" that exposes men to the risks of side effects such as incontinence and erectile dysfunction.

In a meta-analysis of five randomized trials with follow-up periods ranging from ten to twenty years, a prostate cancer mortality reduction was not found (relative risk [RR] 0.96, 95 percent CI 0.85–1.08).[263]

In this meta-analysis of five trials, participants were randomized to control groups or to one-time or repeat screening that occurred at intervals ranging from one to four years. However, the included studies each contained high or unclear risks of bias. The ERSPC trial found a small absolute survival benefit with PSA screening at nine years of follow-up, with an absolute risk reduction of 0.51 per 1,000 men. By sixteen years, the prostate cancer mortality rate in the screening group was 0.53 per 1,000 person-years compared with 0.66 per 1,000 person-years in the control group. The absolute risk reduction of prostate cancer death was 1.76 per 1,000 men, meaning that to avert one prostate cancer death, 570 men needed to be invited to screening, of whom eighteen were expected to be diagnosed with cancer.[264]

Researchers from Weill Cornell Medicine have found that while these efforts have been effective, the incidence of higher-grade disease and metastasis at diagnosis have risen. The research was published on March 22, 2022, in the *Journal of the National Cancer Institute.*

"To our knowledge, this is the first study to demonstrate nationally that low-grade prostate cancer is no longer the most commonly diagnosed type of prostate cancer," said senior author Dr. Jim Hu, the Ronald P. Lynch Professor of Urologic Oncology at Weill Cornell Medicine and director of the LeFrak Center for Robotic Surgery at New York-Presbyterian/Weill Cornell Medical Center.[265]

"One of the weaknesses of PSA/prostate cancer screening was that it led to over-detection of indolent cancers that would not harm men, subjecting them to anxiety and future testing."[266]

In 2012, the US Preventive Services Task Force (USPSTF) recommended against screening all men with the PSA test, concluding that the benefits of the test, which measures levels of a protein often over-produced in prostate cancer cells, did not outweigh the risks. Then in 2018, the USPSTF issued a revision to include shared decision-making for the PSA test for men aged fifty-five to sixty-nine years, reflecting emerging evidence of longer-term benefits and widespread adoption of active surveillance after the detection of low-risk disease.[267]

For their study, Dr. Hu and colleagues identified more than 438,000 men with newly diagnosed prostate cancer between 2010 and 2018 using a nationally representative database. They examined trends in the incidence of prostate cancer by disease risk using several measures. One measure was the Gleason Grade, a pathology score based on the microscopic appearance of the prostate cells, determined at biopsy and after radical prostatectomy, a procedure in which the entire prostate is surgically removed. Additional measures were PSA level and presence of metastasis at diagnosis. They also investigated whether increasing rates of obesity or the advent of newer diagnostic tools such as prebiopsy magnetic resonance imaging (MRI) and biomarkers might explain incidence trends.[268]

The analysis revealed a significant decrease in the incidence of the lowest-risk prostate cancer, Gleason Grade 1 (GG1), falling from fifty-two to twenty-six cases per 100,000 men across all age groups.[269]

"It is encouraging to see that urologists in the United States have moved away from overutilization of radical therapies for the management of low-risk prostate cancer," added author Dr. Leonardo Borregales.[270]

Public health authorities should consider implementing risk-stratified screening, such as MRI or biomarkers, continuing to minimize overdiagnosis and avoid biopsy in men with low-risk prostate cancer while addressing the rising trends of high-grade and metastatic prostate cancer, the authors concluded.[271]

MAYO CLINIC PROCEEDINGS

Fundamental Concepts Regarding Testosterone Deficiency and Treatment

International Expert Consensus Resolutions[272]

Abraham Morgentaler, MD

Michael Zitzmann, MD

Abdulmaged M. Traish, PhD

George Mskhalaya, MD

Claude C. Schulman, MD

Luiz O. Torres, MD

Published: June 21, 2016

When I think of the journey we have been experiencing with testosterone, I think of Prague. Please join me as I *travel down memory lane* to October 1, 2015, when a gathering of many of the most respected physicians in the world convened in Prague, Czech Republic. They were there to develop and publish a worldwide consensus on the medical condition of testosterone deficiency and T therapy. They all knew the clinical importance of this debate and how vital it was to clear the air. They focused on testosterone and men, but we can also apply these findings to women. And incidentally, Barrett Johnson came to me for BHRT the same year.

There is no telling how many lives these physicians have saved by cutting through the myths and providing unanimous resolutions of endorsement for testosterone therapy.

Experts included various medical specialties, including urology, endocrinology, diabetology, internal medicine, and basic science research. In addition to dispelling all the myths surrounding testosterone therapy, nine resolutions were debated and approved unanimously.

> **There is no telling how many lives these physicians have saved by cutting through the myths and providing unanimous resolutions of endorsement for testosterone therapy.**

Unanimously Approved Resolutions[273]

1. Testosterone deficiency (TD) is a well-established, clinically significant medical condition that negatively affects male sexuality, reproduction, general health, and quality of life.

2. Symptoms and signs of TD occur as a result of low levels of T and may benefit from treatment regardless of whether there is an identified underlying etiology.

3. TD is a global public health concern.

4. T therapy for men with TD is effective, rational, and evidence-based.

5. There is no T concentration threshold that reliably distinguishes those who will respond to treatment from those who will not.

6. There is no scientific basis for any age-specific recommendations against the use of T therapy in men.

7. The evidence does not support increased risks of cardiovascular events with T therapy.

8. The evidence does not support increased risk of prostate cancer with T therapy.

9. The evidence supports a major research initiative to explore the possible benefits of T therapy for cardiometabolic disease, including diabetes.

I urge you to read this entire report, available online at Mayo Clinic Proceedings, shown in our citations. If you doubt the science behind BHRT, this unanimous report should clear that up.

I also call your attention to these excerpts from their summary findings:

• "Several resolutions presented in this article contradict recent positions taken by the FDA. It is worth recognizing that although the FDA plays a critical role in the regulation of pharmacotherapeutics, it does not regulate the practice of medicine."

• "Concepts regarding medical issues require medical expertise, which we have attempted to provide in this consensus document. Our group of experts fully endorses the clinical importance of symptoms and signs for men with TD, a concept promoted in medical guidelines but not embraced so far by regulatory agencies."

- "We find no high-quality evidence to support FDA concerns regarding CV (cardio-vascular) risk with T therapy and, to the contrary, find substantial evidence linking low T concentrations to CV disease and mortality, with suggestive evidence of reduced CV risk with T therapy."

- "Moreover, evidence from the recently published Testosterone Trials has itself undermined several FDA recommendations and provided support for our conclusions."

- "These results include the documentation of significant benefits with T therapy, improvement in various TD-related symptoms with treatment, rejection of age-based restrictions on T therapy (men in the Testosterone Trials were all aged 65 years and older), and now level 1 evidence contradicting the assertion that the benefits of T therapy have been adequately confirmed only in men with an identified underlying etiology (classical hypogonadism)."

- "One of the more critical advances in the field has been the identification of the contribution of comorbidities such as diabetes and obesity to TD, which the FDA and other regulatory agencies have so far failed to recognize."[274]

I love watching my patients improve and hearing their stories, and I sincerely wish we could find a way to offer this rejuvenation to everyone.

I have been sharing my thoughts on the most dramatic and phenomenal scientific breakthroughs in medicine that have brought us to this moment. These discoveries have kept me awake at night over the last thirty years. Like frozen moments in time for me, these events bent the arc of healthcare in America and the world, changed the way we think, changed our view of the human body, and that maybe shook up a calcified system from time to time. As you have seen from the groundbreaking studies by brilliant scientists shared in *Restore*, the world is moving faster now. It's a sprint to the Holy Grail.

I'll take you on the next stage of your quest for *optimal wellness*, and that involves your diet, a major piece of this wellness journey. Again, you must choose. And now that you've arrived at this moment in history, you can board the train. The choice is yours. How cool is that? Choose wisely.

The Magnificent Role of Nutrition in Quality of Life—Fasting, Peptides, and Making Good Choices

About a year before I began to write *Restore*, I visited a good friend and colleague in the capital of country music, Nashville, where many of the top authorities in the world in hypertension and heart health practice. I made an appointment to get the advice and counsel of Dr. Mark Houston, author of the recent book *Controlling High Blood Pressure through Nutrition, Nutritional Supplements, Lifestyle, and Drugs* with board-certified nutritionist Lee Bell, NC, BCHN. Also nearby are the clinical offices of another great colleague, Dr. William Seeds, author of *The Peptide Protocols*.

Their book is designed to help prevent and treat high blood pressure and hypertension, the most common primary diagnosis in the United States and a leading cause of heart attack, heart failure, kidney failure, and stroke.

I spent three days of testing with Dr. Mark Houston. (I am really serious about my nutrition.) He is also director of the Hypertension Institute and Vascular Biology and medical director of the Division of Human Nutrition at Saint Thomas Medical Group, Saint Thomas Hospital and Health Services in Nashville, Tennessee. He has published seven books and presented over ten thousand lectures, nationally and internationally, and published over 250 medical articles, and scientific abstracts in peer-reviewed medical journals, books, and book chapters.

Dr. Houston was selected as one of the Top Physicians in Hypertension in the United States in 2008–2018 by the Consumer Research Council, and by *USA Today* as one of the Most Influential Doctors in the United States in both Hypertension and Hyperlipidemia twice in 2009–2010.

While I was testing with him, he suggested I meet with Lee Bell, just down the hall from his office at the Hypertension Institute at Saint Thomas West Hospital Center: "You need to talk with Lee."

Lee Bell, NC, BCHN, is board certified in holistic nutrition, earned a bachelor's degree from the University of Southern California, and graduated from the Bauman College of Holistic Nutrition in Berkeley, California. She is a member of the National Association of Nutrition Professionals (NANP) and the American Association of Nutrition Consultants (AANC). Lee has completed Dr. Ben Lynch's program on methylation and clinical nutrigenomics as well as the Institute for Functional Medicine's Methylation Strategies in the Clinical Management of Depression and Cardiovascular Disease. She holds certification in plant-based nutrition through the T. Colin Campbell Institute at Cornell University and continues her postgraduate education through Harvard Medical School, where she received certification in clinical management of celiac disease.

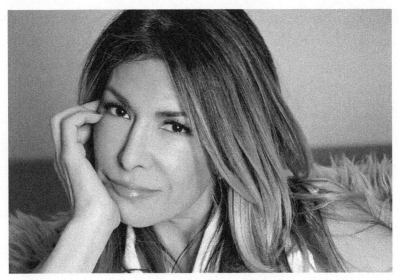

"Lee Bell." Attune Health. Accessed September 1, 2023. https://attunehealth.com/lee-bell-2/.

Lee Bell, NC, BCHN

Lee Bell speaks with authority on the general condition of our food culture in a way I have never heard before. She had so much to say that would be of deep interest to people thinking about BHRT that I share our conversation here.

"People ask me all the time," she said, "what does an optimum human diet look like? I tell them to watch the show on the Discovery Channel called *Naked and Afraid* if you want to see the way humans are supposed to live. Humans are not wired for the steady drip of food all day. Humans are wired to live in a world of scarcity where we don't see food all that much.

"And here really is the rub, or what scientists would call an 'evolutionary mismatch,' that humans are wired to live in a world of scarcity," Lee added.

"The human brain is designed to eat almost every single thing it sees. Because humans, like every other species, are here to propagate the species in order to survive as a species. What happens when you take that very primitive idea of wanting to eat everything, and you move it, not into a world of scarcity, but now it lives in a world of abundance? Now you've got a real problem on your hands."

Lee is very deliberate about her food intake. She regularly fasts and does group "liquid fasts" of seventy-two hours with many of her patients each month.

In January 2020, Lee started with a group of about eight people in Nashville. She would guide them through a seventy-two-hour fluid fast. Again, the differentiator was that it wasn't just water. You could consume sparkling water, tea, or black coffee. Some people would continue to have low-sodium broth in their diet. It was all fluids, but certainly something a little bit more interesting than water. Now eighteen months into that proposition, she reached a hundred people fasting each month with incredible results on their health.

Lee Bell is also a big believer in BHRT.

"You know, hormones, when you think about it from a purely molecular level, are just self-signaling agents like peptides. They just tell the body what to do. What's the primary differentiator as we age? Hormone status."

When we replace those with bioidentical hormone replacement therapies, she says, "People really do notice a profound difference. You have a renewed sense of vitality. And depending on the balance of those hormones, there are a lot of different dials that you can tweak in order to improve the quality of life."

"With respect to fasting, that has been in the American conscious-ness now for about a decade, and we know a lot more about it today. When fasting became adopted by a wide swath of the population, we were able to collect more data about how different strategies or drugs or supplements or peptide therapies, or whatever it is, influence the population. Fasting is an idea that is the *least fadlike idea* that I can come up with. I talk to the patients in our clinic about this all the time, people that are curious about it. I would say five years ago, we had a fair amount of people in the clinic who still hadn't heard of intermittent fasting."

Today, Lee notes, almost everyone that we come across has heard about it, and many of those folks have even tried some iteration of fasting.

There are a lot of different paths to intermittent fasting, she explained, the most popular of which is "what we would call a 16:8, an eight-hour window of opportunity for food or time-restricted eating that we would refer to that."

Fasting has been around since the beginning of time; it's just never been voluntary. It was either due to famine, or it was due to poor crop yield, or it was due to war.

Where intermittent fasting comes into play, does intermittent fasting regulate glucose?

She says it might.

"We used to think that it lowered triglycerides, that it lowered inflammatory status in the body, that it kicked the body into autophagy, which I don't think is true with intermittent fasting, but maybe a longer-term fast."

We now know, Lee said, that the primary benefit of fasting is that when humans confine their meals to a restricted period of time, they consume fewer calories. There's not a tremendous amount of magic to it. It just feels less restrictive than, let's say, diminishing portions, or deciding you were going to aggressively limit the number of calories that you could consume.

Lee tells her patients that there are only three ways to drop body fat. One of them is through intermittent fasting, which leads to a calorie imbalance. The other is limiting the portions of food that we consume, which also leads to a calorie imbalance. Or for some people, they'll limit the certain kinds of foods that they eat. All diets are limiting in some way. The paleo diet restricts carbohydrates. Keto diets do the same. Vegetarianism and veganism limit animal protein.

"The question really becomes where you want to pick your poison in order to create that energy imbalance," she says.

"And for some people, what feels the least restrictive is to say, "Most days I'm going to limit the consumption of food to ten o'clock and six o'clock, or noon and six o'clock, or noon and four o'clock, or I'm going to have one meal a day." All of those are forms of time-restricted eating. As we know today, that is the primary benefit of intermittent fasting. We consume fewer calories; we have a shorter window of opportunity in which to consume meals."

I asked her where she begins with a new patient.

"First and foremost, she said, "I create an individual foundational dietary strategy for anyone I work with. We take into consideration many things, such as age, gender, hormone status, level of activity, health history, and sleep integrity."

In working with the Hypertension Clinic patients, she will come up with things she thinks will work—novelties, if you will.

"I call them recovery strategies," Lee says. "Based on a patient's dietary history, which typically involve struggles, I begin with framing what the challenges might be. In other words, what's the opposition? Is it the management of portions, cravings, emotional eating, the temptation of high-calorie, ultraprocessed foods, lack of support, unrealistic weight-loss expectations?

"First, we have to understand what it means to be human living in a world of abundance. You're going to have to deal with hunger. You're going to have to learn how to deal with cravings. You're going to have to learn how to turn to other options outside of food to find comfort. Maybe it's not legitimate hunger, maybe it's not a craving, maybe it's just the desire to eat.

"That's the nature of the world that we live in because things fundamentally changed in the late 1970s. Prior to that, Americans were really focused on three square meals a day. That was the basic structure of the American diet then."

Lee notes that the big food industry essentially said, "Why bother packaging these gigantic candy bars and bags of chips when we can package them in smaller containers, and we can make them portable, and we can teach the American public that they need snacks to get through the day!"

Prior to that, she reminded me that there really wasn't a whole lot of snacking going on in the United States. That ushered in an era of greater dysregulation with glucose and obesity. And that influenced one of the hormones that keeps us fat: insulin.

Lee explained that insulin became a big subject of curiosity for her about a decade ago, when her youngest son was diagnosed with juvenile diabetes.

"I'm a diabetic educator. But, even for those who don't have type 1 or type 2 diabetes glucose regulation should be an area of concern." According to the Centers for Disease Control (CDC) an estimated 88 million adults over the age of eighteen are prediabetic.[275]

Today, she explained, we have the popularity of GLP-1 receptor agonists, and semaglutides—the class of drugs that were originally conceived for the diabetic population.

"But now we know that a primary attribute is weight loss, that it suppresses appetite, and it does so incredibly well."

"People, again, think there's some magic. *Wow, this is regulating my blood sugar.*"

Well, it is regulating your blood sugar, she explained, but the reason why you're dropping body weight is that this drug affects the satiety center in your brain. This primitive piece we all have to wrestle to the ground now has reinforcements.

> **Now we've got assistance in blunting the hunger dragon.**

"OK, now we've got assistance in blunting the hunger dragon. That's how people ultimately drop body weight on this is that you feel full, very full, very quickly on this class of [*I don't want to call it a drug*] peptide therapy. So it's something that the body recognizes as its own, in the same way that the body would recognize insulin, which was the first peptide ever reproduced. That was in 1920," Lee noted.

IMMUNITY RESIDES IN THE GUT

Over the era of COVID-19, Lee, naturally, frequently got questions about immunity. She found it interesting when she would ask patients if they knew where their immunity resided.

"Now, immunity is a very complex subject, she would say, and it isn't a singular thing. But the gut-associated lymphoid tissue (GALT), which is the largest mass of lymphoid tissue in the body, is in the gut. And so, without optimizing gut health, you can't optimize immunity.

"So that's always the starting place for me. The overwhelming majority of people that I work with have some gut issues. They have inexplicable bloating. They say, 'I have cramping, I have stomach pain. Something just doesn't feel right; I'm constipated all the time; I have loose bowel movements.'"

Lee also thinks this is heavily influenced by stress, one of the challenges of modern life. Stress heavily influences GI function.

"I'm a big proponent of mapping the GI, especially for anybody who suffers from gut issues, there are some extremely sophisticated tests available today. And then once we see that data, we can then compensate for whatever the imbalances may be by knowing if there's overcolonization, an undercolonization of certain kinds of bacteria."

The balance of bacteria in the gut heavily influences everything that has to do with the body. Everything kind of resides in the microbiome.

"I cannot take credit for this analogy," Lee adds, "but the human body is like a symphony. And if any of the systems, whether it's the GI or the circulatory system, or if any of the systems are out of whack, much like in a symphony, if you have a violinist that isn't carrying their musical weight, you're going to hear it. And the same thing happens to the body. Everything influences everything else. The body by nature wants to achieve homeostasis. It likes the idea of everything in balance.

"Dr. Brannon and I agree 100 percent with this: for anybody over the age of 45, the focus of the diet has to be on the avoidance of muscle loss, the avoidance of what we call sarcopenia. I like the idea of a dietary strategy that supports the maintenance of muscle mass.

"I can't stress enough the importance. If you want to stay out of a nursing home, you better maintain muscle mass. And it isn't simply about being able to achieve a lean silhouette. Without muscle, we lose balance. We have differences in glucose regulation. We absolutely need strength in order to maintain vitality as we go through the decades," Lee said.

Lee thinks that we live in a society that's focused too heavily on fat, this almost fat-phobic approach to diet, rather than: "What are the dietary strategies that I can adopt to maintain (at a minimum), and build muscle mass as I go through the decades?"

"Usually, you have to prioritize at least for a short period of time," she explains, one over the other. Either you want to build muscle or want to lose fat, and then later, build muscle. But I would say fasting, depending on how you do it, isn't entirely compatible with muscular hypertrophy. In other words, fasting is not a great strategy for muscle building.

"When somebody comes to me and says, the focus for me for the next three to six months is to lose body fat. I want to be lighter. I want to get some of this weight off my joints. Intermittent fasting would be a fine idea.

"I would say that for somebody who had to resolve to limit their meals to five hours a day, I think it would be a good idea if the goal was to drop body fat, knowing that maybe six months down the line, you shift some of that into a different dietary approach and a different schedule.

"Patients need a lot of support when looking to make permanent change. If you look at the data on weight loss, it's dismal.[276] There's a 95 percent probability for anybody who changes their diet that they will gain their weight back within a five-year period. And of that 95 percent, 83 percent of those will go on to gain more weight than they had to lose, to begin with. So, a big focus of my practice is adopting cutting-edge ideas when it comes to how we can manage what it means to be human.[277]

"For instance, if there's a 95 percent failure rate, what do those five percenters know that have allowed them to maintain their weight loss for over a five-year period? (Which is how we gauge the probability.) You have the highest probability of keeping it off for a lifetime if you can keep it off for five years.

"But you have to think that five years is a long haul. Think about it. You're three years into the same weight. And now, all of a sudden, you're going to see an uptick in body weight. That is common. There are biological reasons for that also."

Lee looks at how her patients can adopt the strategies that go along with a 5 percent lifestyle.

"I deeply agree with Dr. Brannon that the minute humans discovered mortality, they were thinking about how to extend it ... and today, the cutting-edge ideas are not about life span. They're about health span. And I would also argue the fifty, sixty, seventy, eighty, ninety of today is not that of a generation ago, by any stretch of the imagination. There's a lot more air in the ball. We know a lot more. I'd say specifically over the course of the last decade, longevity medicine has really gained exponential knowledge into the aging pathways, and then, what we can do about them.

PEPTIDES

"Recent research indicates that some types of peptides could have a beneficial role in slowing down the aging process, reducing inflammation, and destroying microbes. People may confuse peptides with proteins. Both proteins and peptides are made up of amino acids, but peptides contain far fewer amino acids than proteins," *Medical News Today* describes.[278]

Medical News Today describes peptides as smaller versions of proteins. As supplements, they may have antiaging, anti-inflammatory, or muscle building properties. For this reason, health and cosmetic products often contain different peptides.[279]

This is the first generation in human history that has the choice of how to age. Lee gave us a wonderful word picture of the human body as a symphony. When one instrument gets out of pitch, everyone hears it. That same analogy could be used to describe peptides. Imagine a symphonic orchestra is the human body. Now imagine the Beatles singing backup vocals. That's how we use peptides to make the symphonic homeostasis of the body better.

We want to help you succeed; we'll make sure you can accomplish your goals. It's a way of life, and we will show you the new science that will overturn the apple cart of beliefs that have been wrongly telling us how to keep healthy. We can offer you a structured wellness plan or just a few tips for moving forward. It's up to you. We'll tell you what you should avoid, no matter what. It's your life.

The next thing may be a need to do some repair, and to stimulate your growth hormones. If you're not sleeping well, or you're looking to move to the next level, then I add growth, I add the peptides. If you are recovering from an injury, peptide BPC-157 works great. You can take it locally in a shot. You can also take it orally.

Peptide therapy utilizes natural, effective, and noninvasive supplements to decrease inflammation, help with healing, promote weight loss, hair growth, and healing, and assist in antiaging, contributing to your overall health and well-being.

Some folks may get peptide therapy confused with human growth hormone. They are as different as night and day.

HGH vs. Peptides	Human Growth Hormone	Peptide Therapy
Effects	• Promotes unnatural levels and shuts down natural production • Negatively impacts pituitary function	• Promotes natural release of, as well as natural production, of HGH • Supports pituitary function and health
Safety	• High risk of overdose - levels drop with discontinuation • Many side effects including cancer, elevated cortisol, high blood pressure, and abnormal body enlargement	• Low risk of overdose - production continues after discontinuation • Minimal side-effects such as injection site reactions are possible

Peptides are much safer than human growth hormones and just as effective!

Comparing peptides to human growth hormones brings back memories of the scandals of doping and steroid misuse that plagued professional and amateur sports. Misuse of testosterone and anabolic steroids can lead to steroid use disorder. Steroid use disorder can cause symptoms of sexual dysfunction, mood disorders, and mood swings. Approximately 32 percent of people who misuse anabolic steroids become dependent.[280]

The National Institute on Drug Abuse states clearly that a patient that is dependent on anabolic steroids such as testosterone injections who then transitions to pellet therapy can experience symptoms of withdrawal. Withdrawal symptoms include fatigue, restlessness, loss of appetite, insomnia, decreased libido, steroid cravings, and depression. Withdrawal and elevated estradiol symptoms are similar. Close monitoring of labs and patients' symptoms is necessary to ensure a smooth transition. However, patients with a long-term history of testosterone and anabolic steroid misuse will need ongoing education and guidance to help with the withdrawal phase.[281]

So human growth hormone, while it has been abused, is not necessarily bad. Peptide therapy under the supervision of a physician promotes natural release of this important hormone.

Dr. William Seeds is a phenomenal resource for the advanced use of peptides. His book *The Peptide Protocols* is a classic text.

In the introduction to his book, Dr. Seeds describes how peptides are changing the nature of recovery and of performance and his ten-year history with peptides, first helping "his athlete patients recover faster and then helping them return to the playing field stronger, more agile, and more capable."[282]

In *The Peptide Protocols*, Dr. Seeds notes that perhaps the most paradigm-shifting is that when you look through this powerful lens of the cellular level, you come to realize that peptides offer us a radically new way to define aging. Indeed, aging, as we have come to accept it, is simply cell cycle arrest. Peptides can target this arrest and the reasons for it. "This is a gross simplification, to be sure, but there is great truth in the simplicity of the cell," Dr. Seeds suggests.[283]

Dr. William Seeds takes a close look at the cell cycle, cell behavior, and what happens when cells don't get what they need and begin to morph or make bad decisions. When the cells get to this stage, they become senescent and that's what we are really after with peptides.

By interfering with or stopping cell senescence, when necessary, peptides give us the opportunity to help our patients prevent disease, recover faster, harness aging, and improve overall health. As we advance your health journey, restore your hormones, and regain your body's optimal performance, we may call on peptides from time to time to troubleshoot areas of concern or improve performance.

The music can get better and better from our symphony of instruments and voices. Dr. Seeds consults with doctors around the world in the use of "peptides as adjuvants" that achieve faster, better medical results.[284]

"Peptides offer us nearly miraculous opportunities to change how we treat illness and disease; they also offer us life-changing tools and strategies for preventing disease in the first place. Disease, both chronic and acute, occurs at the level of the cell. Peptides can halt disease by enhancing cell functioning," he says.[285]

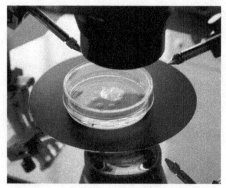

To provide you with a list of peptides currently being deployed by practitioners across the world would be quite lengthy and complicated. Each has protocols, specifically targeting a particular problem.

I turn to the *International Journal of Molecular Science* to keep abreast of the rapidly changing world of peptides. Here's what the journal reported in 2022 regarding the most recent advances in peptide research and its applicability:

"In recent years, peptides have received increased interest in pharmaceutical, food, cosmetics, and various other fields. The high potency, specificity, and good safety profile are the main strengths of bioactive peptides as new and promising therapies that may fill the gap between small molecules and protein drugs."[286]

Journal Authors Cristina Martínez-Villaluenga and Blanca Hernández-Ledesma note that peptides "possess favorable tissue penetration and the capability to engage in specific and high-affinity interactions with endogenous receptors. The positive attributes of peptides have driven research in evaluating peptides as versatile tools for drug discovery and delivery."

The authors also write that in addition, among bioactive peptides, those released from food protein sources "have acquired importance as active components in functional foods and nutraceuticals because they are known to possess regulatory functions that can lead to health benefits."[287]

We deploy peptides to help many patients. If I listed them in *Restore*, the book would be outdated in months because researchers are bursting with new discoveries and uses for peptides. Here is a partial list of some of the applications we currently have fully researched protocols for use in our practice:

- Antiaging
- Fat loss
- Progressive fat loss (enhances fasting)
- Anabolism / enhanced recovery
- Injury healing
- Increase bone growth
- Improve GI recovery
- Improve immune function
- Skin issues

Since the synthesis of the first therapeutic peptide, insulin, in 1921, remarkable achievements have been made resulting in the approval of more than eighty peptide drugs worldwide.[288]

Nature reminds us that the discovery and development of insulin, a peptide with 51 amino acids, has been considered as one of the monumental scientific achievements in drug discovery. The development of peptide drugs has thus become one of the hottest topics in pharmaceutical research. As an example, the article I am sharing about peptides cites 535 recent clinical studies.[289]

Hundreds of peptides are undergoing preclinical studies and clinical development. These peptide drugs have been applied to a wide range of diseases, such as diabetes mellitus, cardiovascular diseases, gastrointestinal diseases, cancer, infectious diseases, and vaccine development.[290]

Hold on to your hats. More is coming every day.

Travel with me down memory lane. No matter what your age, I think you may recall the federal government's food pyramid. We can blame much of today's epidemic of obesity on our leaders' eagerness to tell us how to do everything. In this case, they were wrong. If you have gained weight, it's mostly not your fault. They told us wrong.

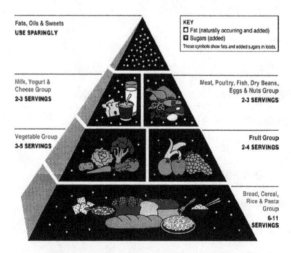

Original (1992) USDA Food Guide Pyramid

THE REASON OUR NATION HAS BECOME OBESE AND UNHEALTHY

The food pyramid traces its roots back to earlier dietary models, such as the dietary circle. In 1972, amid soaring food prices, Sweden's National Board of Health and Welfare developed the idea of "basic foods," both cheap and nutritious, and "supplemental foods" that added nutrition missing from the basic foods. They created a dietary circle model to easily promote these products and their recommended serving sizes to consumers. The United States developed their own dietary circle model, the Basic Seven.

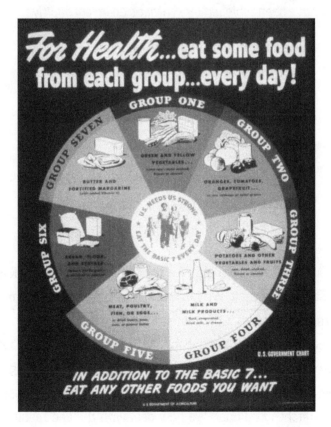

The Basic Seven Dietary Circle, US Department of Agriculture[291]

"DOWN THE RABBIT HOLE"
By Randall Fitzgerald

*The Hundred-Year Lie: How Food and
Medicine Are Destroying Your Health*

> *We are surrounded every day by an invisible
> sea of synthetic chemicals, and our bodies
> absorb them like sponges until we are toxic.*
>
> *We consume foods that have been depleted of
> essential natural healing nutrients. These nutrients
> have been replaced by synthetic chemical additives.*
>
> *These additives in our processed foods interact syn-
> ergistically in our bodies with synthetic chemicals
> absorbed from our water, our air, and our consumer
> products, weakening our immune systems.*
>
> *Once weakened, we become susceptible to
> illnesses and diseases that medical practitioners
> treat with synthetic chemical drug compounds
> that often prove even more toxic to us.*[292]

I explain to every patient who comes in overweight that it is just not their fault. Why in the world do people in the government think that they must tell us what to eat and then embed that into the education system of our children for decades? We used to have eggs and bacon in the morning, a big sandwich at lunch, plenty of healthy meats, and a couple of starches at dinner. We now deal with the end result of sixty years of abiding by our leadership paternalistically telling us exactly how to lead every aspect of our lives. And they miss the target more than they hit it.

> *Ninety percent of the food today was not consumed here a hundred years ago. And 90 percent of the diseases were not here either. Something's going on ...*

The US Department of Agriculture has led us to a society-wide metabolic disorder. Testosterone provides the one thing fighting it. Visceral fat, central obesity, weakening of the muscles—everything works against healthy levels of testosterone.

We increased our sugar intake tremendously. Sixty years ago, fast food did not appear on every street corner. We ate three big meals a day, food high in fat, high in protein, that could actually feed our bodies the proper nutrients. They taught us to go for twelve or so carbohydrates a day; then we created hundreds of thousands of fast-food joints that serve a ridiculous amount of sugar and bread to everyone who drives through.

Our nation had a growing food policy. It shifted from *eating more* following World War II to *eating less* to prevent chronic disease.

In 1977, our Senate Select Committee on Nutrition and Human Needs came out with recommendations. A key influencer was Ancel Keys, PhD, the father of the "Lipid Hypothesis," which blamed fat consumption for heart attacks.

He deployed his own study data to prove his hypothesis. One critic suggested that he had data from twenty-two countries and only used seven. Indeed, well-meaning

Dr. Keys had difficulty finding support in the scientific community, so he turned to accessible politicians. Thus, the pyramid deals with fat as something to avoid while it's OK to eat a lot of bread and pasta.

In 1977, the Ninety-Fifth Congress and the American Society for Clinical Nutrition released *Dietary Goals*. This political emphasis encouraged the consumption of increased amounts of fruits, vegetables, and carbohydrates, and decreased amounts of cholesterol, salt, alcohol, and sugar, as well as fewer eggs.[293]

However, even suggestions that we "eat less" from several agencies became unpopular with food producers because they wanted to continue to sell large quantities of food products and continue generating maximized profit. Subsequently, the USDA provided "gentler" suggestions related to food consumption and faced public investigation after dietary suggestions resulted in decreased sales of many meat products.[294]

In 1991, an effort arose to establish a food pyramid with six food groups. The food industry pushed back on that because "it appeared to make some foods more important both in the shape of the pyramid and in the recommended serving sizes" which had the potential to reduce profits.

So the food industry made it a priority to fight the public introduction by any means possible. A well-orchestrated media attack framed the pyramid as a scheme established by animal rights activists. It then became an agenda from different sectors of the food industry. Nonetheless, the pyramid appeared.[295]

PREVENTION

Well, we do not have a new food pyramid or catchy slogan for how to consume sustenance in the twenty-first century. We know a lot more now. So here are a few tips:

- Rethink *when* you eat.

- Consider intermittent fasting.

- Add protein to your meals.

- Proteins provide essential amino acids in your body that help maintain muscle, skin, and bone health. Furthermore, protein affects the release of hormones ghrelin and leptin, which control appetite.

- Get regular physical exercise.

- Physical exercise helps reduce insulin levels in your body and helps hormone regulation.

- Skip the refined sugar and carbs.

- Keep your sugar and carb levels in check to avoid developing diabetes, obesity, and other diseases.

- Manage stress effectively.

- The two significant hormones affected by stress are cortisol and adrenaline. Try to allocate some time in your day to do things that help reduce your stress levels.

- Consume healthy fats.

- Include high-quality natural fats like fatty fish, avocados, dark chocolate, eggs, and nuts. This helps reduce insulin resistance and appetite and keeps your hormones in check. Avoid seed oils and trans fats (unnatural and the body cannot eliminate them).

- Most importantly, get your hormone levels checked.

- You may have to ask your primary care provider to include the full hormone panel in your next physical but do so.

Two landmark studies occurred in 2016 and 2018 turned the tables on the scientific certainty of dietary impact on cardiovascular disease and mortality.

In 2016, a group of scientists from the Czech Republic used international statistics to search for associational (noncausal) relationships between nutritional factors and the prevalence of cardiovascular disease in forty-two European countries.

The authors concluded:

> Our results do not support the association between cardiovascular disease (CVDs) and saturated fat ... still contained in official dietary guidelines. Instead, they argue with data accumulated from recent studies that link CVD risk with the high glycemic index/load of carbohydrate-based diets. In the absence of any scientific evidence connecting saturated fat with CVDs, these findings show that current dietary recommendations regarding CVDs should be seriously reconsidered.[296]

Then, in November 2017, *Lancet* published the PURE cohort study of the association of fats and carbohydrate intake with cardiovascular disease and mortality in eighteen countries from five continents over seven years:

> High carbohydrate intake was associated with a higher risk of total mortality, whereas total fat and individual

> types of fat were related to lower total mortality. Total fat
> and types of fat were not associated with cardiovascular
> disease, myocardial infarction, or cardiovascular disease
> mortality, whereas saturated fat had an inverse associa-
> tion with stroke. Global dietary guidelines should be recon-
> sidered in light of these findings.[297]

JASON FUNG, MD, AND OCKHAM'S RAZOR

In 2018, Jason Fung, MD, published *The Diabetes Code*, and bril-
liantly uses "Ockham's razor" to simplify the management of type 2
diabetes. Dr. Fung, a trained nephrologist, runs the Intensive Dietary
Management Program at the University of Toronto. William of
Ockham (1287–1347), an English friar and philosopher, postulated
that with complex problems, the hypothesis with the fewest assumptions is usually correct.

Family Medicine reviewer Joseph E. Scherger, MD, MPH,
published an excellent review hailing Dr. Fung's formulation of a new
understanding of obesity by developing the argument that obesity is
a hormonal illness of excess insulin.

"With all food consumption, especially carbohydrates, insulin is
secreted to drive blood sugar into cells. Insulin is, more importantly,
a fat-storage hormone that blocks fat burning and causes excess sugar
to be turned into fat through lipogenesis. Repeatedly eating carbohydrates causes chronically high insulin levels and the steady accumulation of fat,"[298] Dr. Scherger said.

Dr. Fung stresses the importance of fasting to lower insulin levels
enough to begin using body fat for energy. He argues that nutrition
for weight loss has been overly focused on what we eat and not suf-

ficiently focused on how often we eat. Humans have spent most of their time eating just one meal daily.[299]

"Eating three meals a day is cultural and contributes to the epidemic of overweight and obesity, especially with the increased intake of refined carbohydrates,"[300] he emphasized.

In *The Diabetes Code*, Fung furthers this argument to show that insulin resistance causes type 2 diabetes. Doctors have known this for a long time, but Dr. Fung simplifies it for a better understanding of how insulin resistance occurs,[301] Dr. Scherger added.

"The repeated secretion of insulin that causes obesity leads to insulin resistance as a protective mechanism for chronically high insulin levels. This also results in fatty liver early in the disease process—insulin resistance results in the high blood sugar of type 2 diabetes. Overcome insulin resistance, the blood sugar returns to normal, and the type 2 diabetes reverses. Fasting plays a key part in this disease reversal process."[302]

ERECTILE DYSFUNCTION AS AN INDICATOR OF CARDIOVASCULAR DISEASE AND EARLY DEATH

Dr. Merrill Matschke is a urologist. He has over twenty-five years of experience in urology and specializes in male reproductive medicine and surgery. He's leading the development of the men's health program at Advocate Aurora Health, a large Midwestern healthcare system.

His theory has a lot to do with men's health and especially erectile dysfunction:

> You start to get problems with decreased nitric oxide production," from atherosclerosis, decreased blood flow, and

> low T—which is a huge interest of mine because testos-
> terone, when it's low, does not allow nitric oxide scent to
> work correctly. It is an androgen-dependent enzyme, and
> it has been well-described and proven. Low T, which is a
> huge part of my practice, is a common denominator. All
> these things intersect. When that happens, the tissues do
> not do well.[303]

Men especially need to understand what's happening to their own body, he explains, and if their T is low, if they have diabetes, if they have neuropathy from it, one of the things they're going to start not to have happen are nighttime erections.

When we get nighttime erections, Dr. Matschke explains that it's actually a preventative maintenance mechanism to maintain the health of the smooth muscle tissue inside the penis. That tissue needs high oxygen exposure on a regular basis, or else it's going to start to go through the process of apoptosis and conversion from smooth muscle to collagen.[304]

"This tissue is probably the most exquisitely sensitive tissue to low oxygen tension in the body. It is the canary in the coal mine, it's the check engine light, it is the thing we should be listening to,"[305] Dr. Matschke adds.

"When you see T come down, this impacts the efficiency of nitric oxide production. You're now promoting endothelial dysfunction. I often tell my patients, 'ED equals ED equals ED: erectile dysfunction equals endothelial dysfunction equals early death.' I try to tie it all together."[306]

Dr. Matschke notes that "low T is a bigger deal than I think we realize." [307]

I agree. Take diabetes, for example.

Diabetes and Testosterone Therapy

"I have been trying to educate endocrine system providers with the data out of Europe on long-term testosterone replacement in people with type 2 diabetes with low T and ED," he adds. "As you replace T in these men, not only are you seeing improvements in all their markers of insulin resistance and sensitivity, but you're also curing a higher percentage of type 2 diabetes,"[308] Dr. Matschke says.

He points to a recent study. It was a long-term, real-world, eleven-year clinic-based study: "Remission of type 2 diabetes following long-term treatment with injectable testosterone undecanoate in patients with hypogonadism and type 2 diabetes: 11-year data from a real-world registry study."[309]

It looked at hundreds of men with diabetes and low T. Half of them took T, and the other half did not. They've been following these men for eleven years, he explained. After eleven years, 34 percent of the men treated with testosterone were no longer diabetic, and most of these men had improved measures of A1C, fasting plasma glucose, and fasting insulin, he noted.[310]

That single-site study, conducted in Bremerhaven, Germany, found that testosterone therapy reversed type 2 diabetes in a one-third of the study participants.[311]

Barbara Branning of the University of Buffalo News Center, prepared a news release entitled "UB Diabetes Expert's Research Shows Testosterone Therapy Can Lead to Remission in Men with Type 2 Diabetes."[312]

The study was cowritten by Paresh Dandona, MD, PhD, SUNY distinguished professor in the Department of Medicine in the Jacobs School of Medicine and Biomedical Sciences at UB.

The study finds the male hormone reversed the condition in one-third of clinical trial participants:

> The occurrence of this syndrome is common and with appropriate testosterone replacement, obesity insulin resistance and diabetes may be reversible," said Paresh Dandona, MD, PhD, SUNY Distinguished Professor in the Department of Medicine in the Jacobs School of Medicine and Biomedical Sciences at UB. He co-authored the study, titled "Remission of type 2 diabetes following long-term treatment with injectable testosterone undecanoate in patients with hypogonadism and type 2 diabetes: 11-year data from a real-world registry study.[313]

The prospective, registry-based study was published in the online journal *Diabetes, Obesity and Metabolism*. Dr. Dandona also presented the data to the Annual Mohan Diabetes Foundation Symposium in Chennai, India, where he was given the organization's Lifetime Achievement Award.

NUTRIENT DEFICIENCIES

Joseph M. Mercola, MD, a multiple *New York Times* best-selling author and osteopathic physician, offers the most clearly articulated information I have seen on nutrients and wellness. He is a board-certified health activist and founder of a robust natural health website. Dr. Mercola's provocative work and "question everything" philosophy has elicited debate from the medical and nonmedical community alike. He suggests that the most common nutrient deficiencies include vitamin D, magnesium, vitamin K2, carnosine (beta-alanine), and vitamin B12.[314]

These are some of the first things we look at when blood chemistry results arrive. Your body depends on essential nutrients for growth, development and health maintenance, and deficiencies in certain vitamins can impact your immunity, vision, wound healing, bone health, and much more.

"Neurological damage is possible from lack of vitamin B12, for instance, while vitamin A deficiency can lead to night blindness," he observes.[315]

"If you wait until the symptoms show, you could be in deep trouble," Dr. Mercola warns. These nutrients are essential for your health and for preventing numerous diseases including diabetes, heart disease and cancer,[316] he says.

PREVENTING ALZHEIMER'S THROUGH TIME-RESTRICTED EATING

Dr. Mercola is a big believer in fasting. Among the many benefits of time-restricted eating, he explains, is the "upregulation of autophagy and mitophagy—natural cleansing processes necessary for optimal cellular renewal and function."

"The cycling of feasting (feeding) and famine (fasting) mimics the eating habits of our ancestors and restores your body to a more natural state that allows a whole host of biochemical benefits to occur. It's a powerful approach that not only facilitates weight loss, but also helps reduce your risk of chronic diseases like Type 2 diabetes, heart disease, cancer, and Alzheimer's,"[317] Dr. Mercola notes.

Dr. Mercola points to a January 2020 review research paper, where researchers explain how caloric restriction helps combat Alzheimer's specifically, through these autophagy pathways.

As explained in "The Effects of Caloric Restriction and Its Mimetics in Alzheimer's Disease through Autophagy Pathways,"[318] two of the pathology hallmarks of Alzheimer's are amyloid beta plaques and neurofibrillary tangles formed by aggregates of tau protein.

"The aberrant accumulation of these misfolded and aggregated proteins results in neurotoxicity, and AD is therefore recognized as a proteinopathy," the paper states. In other words, they occur when there's insufficient autophagy occurring in your body. The good news is you can upregulate autophagy, and one of the simplest ways is by implementing time-restricted eating.[319]

I follow an intermittent fasting schedule, where I fast for 18 hours and have a 6-hour window for eating. My diet primarily consists of abundant animal protein, animal fats, and free-range eggs as its core components.

Our team has developed some very concise communications to help our patients evaluate their eating habits. I include these to summarize my thinking on the vital importance of diet.

DIET AS A MEANS TO PREVENT CANCER AND EVEN REVERSE PROGRESSION - *BENEFICIAL*

- **Ketogenic diet or diet of organic, plant-based, Whole Foods** (unprocessed plant foods) — "rainbow diet" — reduces insulin levels

- **Cruciferous vegetables** — boost the activity of detoxifying enzymes in the liver; have 3+ servings/week

- **Fiber** — controls blood sugar and decreases estrogen levels

- **Intermittent fasting** (e.g., 8 hours fed, 16 hours fasted) to reduce insulin levels

- **Grass-fed, grass-finished, pasture-raised beef** — ate nothing but grass their entire lives; higher in omega-3 fatty acids, conjugated linoleic acids (a "good" omega-6), vitamin E, vitamin A; minimally cooked, in a ration of 1:5 with plant-based food volume

- **Flaxseeds** – contain both essential omega-3 fatty acids plus lignan (lignans are phytoestrogens that can dampen the effects of estrogen); lowers cancer proliferation rate; increase rate of cancer cell clearance; 3 tablespoons/day

- **Walnuts** – suppress cancer cell growth in vitro; prevent cancer deaths (PREDIMED study); high in antioxidants and omega-3 fats; 3 oz/day

"Nutrition is life serving whereas pharmaceuticals are mitochondrial poison."

—MARK SIRCUS, AC., OMD, DM (P)

PROFESSOR OF NATURAL ONCOLOGY, DA VINCI INSTITUTE OF HOLISTIC MEDICINE

DOCTOR OF ORIENTAL AND PASTORAL MEDICINE

FOUNDER OF NATURAL ALLOPATHIC MEDICINE

The Costs and Minor Side Effects of BHRT

I deeply wish we could find a way to offer this rejuvenation to everyone. The one thing we can do is to keep the charges down. Still, we must run a medical practice and pay good people to enjoy their careers here. But I want great American heroes, and average citizens, men and women of all ages, to be able to access this miracle, to conclude that the cost is worth it, not excessive, and most of all, fair and uninhibited by insurance policies.

For example, our fees are currently set to annually average out to about $4 to $7 per day for a man and slightly less for a woman. At the time of this book's publication, our practice asks for a modest one-time-in-your-life consulting fee. You will never get charged again for my advice. Our philosophy is to make this therapy as affordable as possible, giving people a choice. For example, many folks spend several bucks a day on fancy coffee or incidentals. That's a choice, then. Do I buy that fancy coffee or get BHRT that will impact me for the rest of my life?

You most definitely can find other providers that charge a lot more than this. But you probably will not find many who charge less. And we're able to do this without the interference of insurance companies, which in my opinion, always raise costs so they can take their share and remove independent decision-making from doctors. And we need to nurture this movement without the help of a government medical-industrial complex that has grown too big to be of any use.

I refuse to overcharge for this stunning, breakthrough remedy to the ills of aging. I would not champion this if only rich people could afford it.

Unfortunately, the opposite seems to be going around. The *New York Times* published a report in February 2023 from researchers at Brigham and Women's Hospital in Massachusetts,[320] which found that the median price of a new drug was around $180,000 in 2021, up from $2,100 in 2008.[321]

"Those high prices are a factor in a stark wealth gap in medical outcomes," the *New York Times* continued. Dr. Otis Brawley, a professor of oncology and epidemiology at Johns Hopkins University, points to cancer, where "the death rate for Americans with college educations, a proxy for wealth, is 90.9 per 100,000 per year. For those with a high school education or less, the rate is 247.3."[322]

The New York Times authors Gina Kolata and Francesca Paris add that out-of-pocket costs can run to thousands or tens of thousands of dollars. "Often, even those who can afford commercial health coverage or get it through their employer may face insurers that refuse to pay. Other times, an insurer pays part of the cost, but high co-pays, deductibles, and cost-sharing put treatments out of reach for many."[323]

Some doctors agonize over balancing effective treatments with anxieties about the financial burdens on their patients. We're not going to be among them.

After BHRT, if our patients want to engage our wellness team in extended counseling, we have a structured program available for a modest fee. Our team will go in depth with you on how and what you eat, where you think you're healthy, and where you're not, and coach you about fasting. We make this as inexpensive as possible and as simple as possible. We know that if we prescribe a list of forty things for you to change, it will not work. This program is tailored for BHRT patients as well as non-BHRT patients who are fighting obesity, thyroid problems, or other chronic issues.

MINOR SIDE EFFECTS OF BHRT

Having performed bioidentical hormone replacement using pellets for thousands of patients, both men and women, we know that these pellets are gentle, natural products, which, ironically, have quite powerful effects.

BHRT is not a cure-all. It returns your hormones to the best or most favorable levels for your body, so it can function the way it should.

You will still age, but you will age gracefully, as you were designed to. BHRT is about giving your body an internal advantage to help cope with growing older.

While no research shows any life-threatening or long-term dangers from this therapy, I want all my patients to be aware of minor side effects. Pellets are typically very well tolerated. Many of these side effects will occur in the first month while the body is adjusting to the new hormone levels but then diminish over time.

Be aware; not all patients will experience these side effects. Some patients may experience none, and some may only experience one or two. However, in the spirit of full disclosure, we list every possible side effect of BHRT so you can adequately weigh the risks versus the benefits.

Minor Pain during Pellet Placement

There can be some minor pain during the pellet placement procedure, which happens every four to six months, depending on your blood test results. Typically, this pain only lasts a few seconds while injecting the lidocaine. It feels similar to a bee sting. The actual pellet insertion is nearly painless, though you may feel some slight pressure. We have worked diligently over the last decade to make this process better and less uncomfortable. You will be surprised at how quickly and efficiently this is done.

Minimal Hair Thinning or Loss

The American Academy of Dermatology says that as we age, both men and women lose fifty to one hundred hairs a day as a normal fact of life.[324] Hormone replacement, at times, speeds that up.

We informally keep track of the hair loss reports from our patients. About 2 to 4 percent of my patients (both men and women) do experience some hair thinning.

Unfortunately, some people will experience one of these two side effects of testosterone supplementation. If either of these occurs for you, you can take steps to minimize it in the future.

We recommend biotin b7, and the supplement saw palmetto as effective hair loss remedies. We also like a product called Collagenics, another alternative for hair loss prevention that works well for our patients, as do copper-containing peptides.

Mild Acne

Another 1 to 3 percent of my patients have experienced mild acne breakouts, which are treatable with over-the-counter acne medications and are not a long-term issue. Usually, acne will lessen over time with continued treatments. Patients who experience this side effect sometimes say they don't mind breaking out like a teenager because they also have the energy, stamina, and sex drive of a teenager!

Minor Facial Hair Growth

Testosterone can sometimes stimulate facial hair growth, which is not something that bothers men (most don't even notice), but in our experience, about 2 to 5 percent of women it affects, it can be bothersome.

Several options for solving this problem include electrolysis, waxing, laser hair removal, bleaching, shaving, or a medication called spironolactone, which blocks skin five-alpha-reductase and can thin hair. If you experience this side effect, we can discuss the option that would be best for you.

Other Minor Side Effects for Women

Women who receive estrogen will experience a slight enlargement of their breasts, as well as a slightly larger clitoris. I have found some women like it, some don't mind one way or another, and some are unhappy with the side effect. A slightly larger clitoris is due to testosterone supplementation. For some women, the clitoris will shrink back to its original size with continued pellet therapy; for others, it will remain slightly larger. The critical thing to note is that it will not continue to grow after its first initial growth spurt during the first month or two. It will remain the same size as you continue therapy over the years.

Voice Deepening

Some women or men may experience a slight voice deepening due to testosterone therapy. It is so subtle that it is usually not noticeable to anyone but the patient.

Conception

Testosterone therapy suppresses the development of sperm; therefore, it is not recommended for men trying to conceive with a partner. Current research shows that sperm counts return to normal after pellet therapy is discontinued, should the patient decide to have children. (There are ways to increase sperm count and continue BHRT with agents that may include injectable gonadotropins, selective estrogen receptor modulators, and aromatase inhibitors.)[325]

BHRT should not, under any circumstances, be used as a method of contraception. A man will still have viable sperm on BHRT, just not as many.

A Decrease in Testicular Size for Men

Testosterone suppresses natural testosterone production in the testes. BHRT, in essence, does the work *for* your body, or over time, this could result in a decrease in the size of a man's testicles. The size decrease is reversible. If BHRT is discontinued, the testicles will return to their previous size. For most men, it is not an issue, but it's a side effect we want patients to be aware of.

Higher Red Blood Cell Counts for Men

Men given bioidentical testosterone will experience increases in strength and energy levels, partly due to a proliferation of red blood cells and the extra hemoglobin that carries oxygen to all the cells in higher numbers.

Critics of BHRT speculate that an elevated red blood cell mass increases the risk of blood clots and strokes. That fear is unfounded as professional athletes whose hemoglobin counts are as high as 24 grams per deciliter do not experience cardiovascular events."

However, as a precautionary measure, when a patient's red blood cell count becomes higher than the normal range (erythrocytosis), we resolve the issue by either decreasing his testosterone a little or recommending he donate blood about every four months. Simply donating blood will allow his red blood cell count to return to normal.

Breast Enlargement for Men

In male patients, the body will naturally convert excess testosterone to estrogen, which can result in the growth of fatty tissue around the pectoral muscles, also known as gynecomastia, which occurs rarely, primarily to those who are genetically disposed.

To avoid this, we recommend that all our male patients take DIM. This supplement helps metabolize excess estrogen; it is enough for most men. However, a few patients may require a prescription medication called Letrozole, an aromatase inhibitor that we use off-label for estrogen control. (When a medication is used in a so-called off-label manner, all that means is that it is used to treat a condition other than the specific one for which the Food and Drug Administration originally approved it.)

If any of these side effects sound like something that would outweigh the benefits of BHRT, I suggest you do some additional research and take more time with your decision. *Informed consent* is an essential part of our practice. That means we will make every effort to ensure the patient understands the purpose, benefits, and risks of pellet therapy ahead of time. We will endeavor to ensure the patient is well-educated, with the information presented both orally and in writing. That is the foundation of ethical medicine.

Let me emphasize that the side effects are mild because we keep your hormones at the correct physiological levels. When you compare them to the much more severe side effects that may accompany synthetic hormone treatments (high cholesterol, obesity, heart attacks, strokes, dementia, cancer, and other diseases that bioidentical hormones have proven to prevent), it is easy to see why so many people choose BHRT.

Pellet Expulsion

Typically, a man will receive anywhere from six to twelve pellets at a time, depending on his lab levels. His pellets will contain bioidentical testosterone, with each pellet having a dosage of 200 mg. The dosage amount is based upon a precise mathematical algorithm individualized for each person.

The pellets we use for women are a bioidentical testosterone pellet and an estrogen pellet. Depending on their lab work, all our female patients receive somewhere between 75 to 150 mg of testosterone and somewhere between 6 to 25 mg of estrogen. In some instances, if women are still ovulating or have a tendency toward estrogen dominance, they may receive no estrogen at all. Each patient's case is evaluated carefully to determine the best course of action for her as an individual.

We try to minimize the rate of expulsion as much as possible. For women, the rate is very low, about one in a thousand. We're proud of the fact that our accidental expulsion rate is only approximately 1 percent for men and .1 percent for women.

We do recommend that patients refrain from vigorous physical activity, particularly on the first day, but also for up to five days after your placement. If you have little body fat, you will have a higher likelihood of this happening, so lean individuals should be extracareful during this time.

Men need to be extracareful because they receive more pellets than women. If one of your pellets is expelled, you will see the pellet when you remove your bandage. It will look like a tiny white cylindrical object like a long grain of white rice. It is always a good idea to remove your bandage carefully and check for any expulsions. You will need to look closely.

So what happens if a pellet is expelled? Simply call to come back in and reinsert a replacement pellet.

WHO SHOULD NOT TAKE BIOIDENTICAL HORMONES?

Pellets are not recommended for the following people:

- Patients who have a yam allergy.

- Women who are pregnant or wish to become pregnant within three months.

- Men who want to impregnate their partner within three months.

- Any woman who currently has cancer or who has been treated for cancer. A delay of five years is advised for breast cancer and two years for uterine cancers. Shared decision-making is a reasonable approach for BHRT use in symptomatic breast cancer survivors.

- Males should delay BHRT for one year following prostate cancer when genetic predisposition is not involved.

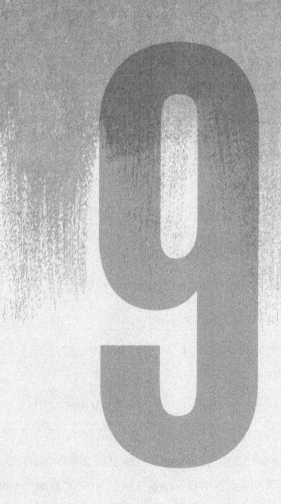

There's Never Been a Time Like This in Human Health

T hose of us who have restored our hormones know what's behind us. By "behind us," I mean that there is a lot of worry in the rearview mirror. We know that our higher hormone level gives us a better chance at facing down the relentless frailty of aging, leading a life with energy and zest for life. That's the path we have taken. We have chosen well to take a shot at this restoration.

We've shown you the beauty of this new restoration journey we now find ourselves considering. The cub grows into a lion. The swan was the ugly duckling. The complete journey of a woman through her stages of life. A young boy growing up to become a man. All of us wishing and praying for strength and dignity when we grow old.

After our first BHRT, we feel a lot better. Many of our low hormone symptoms are diminished. Our chances of encountering osteoporosis, cancer, or heart disease are less now. The number-one cause of death for men and women over sixty-five is falling down.[326] Even if these threats arise at our door, our bodies are now more robust. We sleep better. Our diet is better. We're getting more exercise. Our mood is brightened.

A brief glance in the rearview mirror reminds us that we have left a lot behind us. Good riddance to the brain fog and tiredness, rotten moods, poor motivation, insufficient sleep, lack of stamina, diminished libido, weakened bones, and shuttered sex life.

The path we have been on has been one we chose. We didn't ask anyone for permission. We did not ask our insurance company. We did not phone the federal government, the state government, or our local elected leadership. We made the call. We did not ask our skeptical friends. We decided to safely restore our bodies. The whistle has blown, the game is back on, and we're in that game 100 percent.

There has never been a generation on this planet in recorded history that has had this choice in how we age. Ever. That one realization, or awakening, takes a while to set in. We can do this.

THE QUEST OF THE GRAIL: ON THE EVE
By Ernest Rhys (Author)

Lays of the Round Table and Other Lyric Romances, 1905

I

"Before you take this Quest," (he said), 'in order set, —

Each knight around the Table, —come, sup with me yet;

Come, keep the feast, that after us men never shall forget!'

II

Now, round the Table seated, each tall knight in his place,

Hears noises like to thunder, and sees a light whose rays

Make shine his fellows by him, with brows more bright than day's.

III

Not one could speak, for wonder. Then lo, within the hall

Wrapt round with snow-white samite,
the blessed Sancgreal

And sweetest savours filled the board;
and meat and drink for all.

IV

The mystic Vessel like a gleam went by: it could not stay:

And the knights all fell to feasting,
and the vision passed away,

That all shall quest, but few shall find,
until the earth's last day.[327]

The mystic vessel went by. Tragically in this story, the noble and chivalrous Knights of the Round Table never figured it out.

The Holy Grail has never been found. Millions believe it's still out there. Countless souls looked for the Fountain of Youth, looking for restoration. They were all looking for a way to make the deterioration stop. Like buying a lottery ticket, they have been looking for hope, a chance to *restore* their health.

I hope that you felt something when reading *Restore*. I hope you appreciate the science behind this breakthrough and the devoted physicians and researchers who have dedicated their careers to putting the puzzle together.

You may have felt another sensation, perhaps in a quiet moment. Maybe at some point in reading our narrative, you thought about what it might be like to take that journey. Whether you are eighteen or eighty, that's your question to ask. *I have one life. Do I want to live it fully?*

Here it is. Our moment of perfect clarity. We now understand we have a new freedom. We can choose a healthcare product that can revolutionize our aging process and begin to experience vitality in old age that has never been available to people before this point in history. That, my friends, is the moment of arrival. The moment of becoming *free*. Here comes the sun. The knights felt this as they bid their king goodbye and once again felt the joy and liberty of a grand quest.

> **Whether you are eighteen or eighty, that's your question to ask. *I have one life. Do I want to live it fully?***

One can be consumed with fear of taking responsibility for one's life, but nothing compares to the feeling of liberty when you do so. Freedom over coercion. Liberty over compulsion. Your quest and its rewards await.

Now your hormone levels are like a twenty-five-year-old again, and you have the accumulated knowledge and wisdom of your years. To me, that's the Holy Grail. The Holy Grail is having your *health and life span* occupy the same real estate. For me, that's all we can ever ask for in this life.

I named this book *Restore*. Initially, it represented a perfect name for the BHRT experience. Our hormones fade as we age, so we choose to restore them. Then as I thought about it, the name works on many levels: restoring the dream of youthful strength and a zest for life while retaining the wisdom of aging. That's a universal hope.

> **The Holy Grail is having your *health and life span* occupy the same real estate.**

We're restoring our spirit of curiosity, our hope, and our passion for humanity.

We're, in a sense, restoring our youthful outlook. Choosing wisely. I will never forget the epic Grail Knight scene in *Indiana Jones and the Last Crusade*.

The Grail Knight is willing to give up the Holy Grail to Indiana Jones. But he must choose from an array of similar cups.

"You must choose," he tells Indiana. "But choose wisely."

We are joining up with millions who, by our choices, are shoving America's episodic sick-care healthcare system into a future that embraces prevention, no longer as an afterthought. There's a seat for each of us at this grand round table.

We're restoring our belief in the power of medical science, the evidence-based pursuit of new ideas, or old ideas made better by innovation. Not old ideas held onto too long by Big Pharma. Not the old idea of asking the permission of our government, or worse, our insurance company, ready and willing to tell us exactly how to lead our lives to their best financial advantage.

We're restoring our belief in ourselves.

The three most incredible blessings in life are not recognized while you have them but only after you've lost them, such as your health, youth, and freedom. All three are connected. There is great freedom in taking charge of your health. The benefits impact the quality of your entire life.

Those who are free know how to say: You know what? *I'm* doing this. We'll see what happens. I'm not going to blame anybody but myself. I love that. What's wrong with owning that responsibility? Based on my own experience and the data I've gathered through the years, thousands of patients had no severe complications and there was an overall 98 percent satisfaction rate. That clears the way for this dream, our modern-day mystical vessel that is enchanting just to think about.

The most frequent words I hear every day are *I wish I had done it sooner.* How often have you seen an eighty-year-old man or woman decide to be a marathon runner or have someone start a business at eighty? Go to a Rolling Stones concert; their average age is seventy-six. And this is not a $100,000 stem cell procedure or new medicine that costs $8,000 a month. We have enough of those.

BHRT costs about as much as a nice upscale cup of coffee every day. Everyone has a seat at this table.

My wife, Jody, and I have transformed our lives with BHRT. This restoration is quite real, and it keeps getting better every day. We don't even think about aging anymore. We have enormous energy and passion for our calling.

And this joy keeps being sent back to us from grateful patients. Like knights who rode the lands on their crusade, we have restored the ability of our followers to cross the winter seas, meet difficult challenges, meet every day with new energy and passion, seek what they want their lives to be, and perhaps most significantly, to express their personal freedom and shed the need to ask permission to heal and restore their vitality. I call that *restoration.*

Thank you for sharing my journey. In sincere gratitude and love, here's my humble parting gift to you, dear reader: a suggested affirmation, a promise to yourself and your family:

> I stand on my freedom to choose wisely. I choose not to grow old with brittle bones, to not age with constant chronic illness, and to not accept the fact that I must become lesser intellectually or physically than I am today. I will restore the strength of my sexuality. I will not accept my government telling me what I should eat, how I should care for my body chemistry, or what measures I have permission to take to survive this journey as a vital human

being. To my bloated government, and to my friends in the once-noble insurance industry, thank you for your interest. I'll take it from here.

I love freedom.

Dr. Greg Brannon and his Optimal Bio practice can easily be contacted by going to https://optimalbio.com/

Optimal Bio has nine locations
throughout the nation at time of publication.

Other Books and Research to Inspire You

The Hormone Handbook: Optimizing Your Health through Bioidentical Hormones
By Greg Brannon, MD, FACOG
2020

Outlive: The Science & Art of Longevity
By Peter Attia, MD
2023

Ageless: The Naked Truth about Bioidentical Hormones
By Suzanne Somers
2007

If I Understood You, Would I Have This Look on My Face?: My Adventures in the Art and Science of Relating and Communicating
By Alan Alda
2017

Sex Hormones in Neurodegenerative Processes and Diseases
By Gorazd Drevenšek, MSc, PhD
2018

Testosterone for Life: Recharge Your Vitality, Sex Drive, Muscle Mass, and Overall Health

By Abraham Morgentaler, MD, FACS
2008

*Estrogen Matters: Why Taking Hormones in Menopause Can Improve
Women's Well-Being and Lengthen Their Lives—Without Raising the
Risk of Breast Cancer*
By Carol Tavris, PhD, and Avrum Bluming, MD
2018

*The Definitive Testosterone Replacement Therapy Manual: How to
Optimize Your Testosterone for Lifelong Health and Happiness*
By Jay Campbell
2015

Lies My Gov't Told Me: And the Better Future Coming
By Robert Malone, MD, MA
2023

Ageless: The New Science of Getting Older Without Getting Old
By Andrew Steele, PhD
2022

Hormone Optimization in Preventive/Regenerative Medicine
By Ron Rothenberg, MD, Kris Hart, MN, FNP, RN-C, and
Roger Rothenberg, BA
2012

Feel Younger, Stronger, Sexier: The Life-Saving TRUTH about Bioidentical Hormones
By Dr. Dan Hale
2015

The Law
By Frédéric Bastiat
1850

A Voice to America: The Present Crisis in the United States
By Thomas Bangs Thorpe
1855

The Hundred-Year Lie: How Food and Medicine Are Destroying Your Health
By Randall Fitzgerald
2006

Fast This Way: Burn Fat, Heal Inflammation, and Eat Like the High-Performing Human You Were Meant to Be
By Dave Asprey
2021

What to Eat When: A Strategic Plan to Improve Your Health & Life through Food
By Michael F. Roizen, MD, and Michael Crupain, MD, MPH
2019

The Slow Moon Climbs: The Science, History, and Meaning of Menopause
By Susan P. Mattern
2019

Controlling High Blood Pressure through Nutrition, Nutritional Supplements, Lifestyle, and Drugs
Dr. Mark Houston with Board Certified Nutritionist Lee Bell, NC, BCHN
2020

The Peptide Protocols
By William A. Seeds, MD
2020

"New Research Shows Men with Low Testosterone Are More Likely
to Die from COVID-19"
2021
https://scitechdaily.com/new-research-shows-men-with-low-testosterone-are-more-likely-to-die-from-covid-19/?utm_source=TrendMD&utm_medium=cpc&utm_campaign=SciTechDaily_TrendMD_0

"Biomarker Discovered That Predicts Type 2 Diabetes Many Years
Before Diagnosis"
2021
https://scitechdaily.com/biomarker-discovered-that-predicts-type-2-diabetes-many-years-before-diagnosis/?utm_source=TrendMD&utm_medium=cpc&utm_campaign=SciTechDaily_TrendMD_0

"A Quick and Easy Scan Is a Reliable Predictor of Dementia"
2022
https://scitechdaily.com/a-quick-and-easy-scan-is-a-reliable-predictor-of-dementia/?utm_source=TrendMD&utm_medium=cpc&utm_campaign=SciTechDaily_TrendMD_0

"Severe Depression Affects Women and Men Differently—Scientists May Have Finally Discovered Why"
2022
https://scitechdaily.com/severe-depression-affects-women-and-men-differently-scientists-may-have-finally-discovered-

why/?utm_source=TrendMD&utm_medium=cpc&utm_
campaign=SciTechDaily_TrendMD_0

"Scientists Discover How Sex Hormones Define Brain Differences
between Men and Women"
2022
https://scitechdaily.com/scientists-discover-how-sex-
hormones-define-brain-differences-between-men-and-
women/?utm_source=TrendMD&utm_medium=cpc&utm_
campaign=SciTechDaily_TrendMD_0

"PTA: Low Testosterone and Male Hypogonadism"
2021
https://www.uspharmacist.com/article/low-testosterone-
and-male-hypogonadism?utm_source=TrendMD&utm_
medium=cpc&utm_campaign=US_Pharmacist_TrendMD_1

"Testosterone Levels Can Predict and Treat Diseases. But How Do
You Determine Your 'Right Level'?"
https://geneticliteracyproject.org/2019/06/27/testosterone-levels-
can-predict-and-treat-diseases-but-how-do-you-determine-your-
right-level/?utm_source=TrendMD&utm_medium=cpc&utm_
campaign=Genetic_Literacy_Project_TrendMD_1

"A Marker of Leydig Cell Function and Testis-Bone-Skeletal Muscle
Network"
https://www.eurekaselect.com/article/110228?utm_
source=TrendMD&utm_medium=cpc&utm_campaign=Protein_
Pept_Lett_TrendMD_1

"HIV-Associated Wasting Prevalence in the Era of Modern Antiret-
roviral Therapy"
2022

https://journals.lww.com/aidsonline/Fulltext/2022/01010/HIV_
associated_wasting_prevalence_in_the_era_of.14.aspx?utm_
source=TrendMD&utm_medium=cpc&utm_campaign=AIDS_
TrendMD_1

"Low Testosterone Means a High Risk of Severe COVID-19 for Men"
https://scitechdaily.com/
low-testosterone-means-high-risk-of-severe-covid-19-for-men/

"Study Finds That Testosterone Promotes 'Cuddling'"
https://scitechdaily.com/
study-finds-that-testosterone-promotes-cuddling/

"New Research Shows Men with Low Testosterone Are More Likely
to Die From COVID-19"
https://scitechdaily.com/new-research-shows-men-with-low-
testosterone-are-more-likely-to-die-from-covid-19/

"Testosterone Drives the Dark Side of Success: Meerkat Societies
Fall Apart When Aggression Is Taken Away"
https://scitechdaily.com/testosterone-drives-the-dark-side-of-suc-
cess-meerkat-societies-fall-apart-when-aggression-is-taken-away/

"Lower Testosterone During Puberty Increases the Brain's Sensitivity to the Sex Hormone in Adulthood"
https://scitechdaily.com/lower-testosterone-during-puberty-
increases-the-brains-sensitivity-to-the-sex-hormone-in-adulthood/

"Low-Calorie Ketogenic Diet Can Help Testosterone Levels in
Overweight Men"
https://scitechdaily.com/low-calorie-ketogenic-diet-can-help-
testosterone-levels-in-overweight-men/

"New Evidence for Using Testosterone Therapy to Treat Obesity—
Mean Weight Loss of 50 Pounds"
https://scitechdaily.com/new-evidence-for-using-testosterone-
therapy-to-treat-obesity-mean-weight-loss-of-50-pounds/

"Hormone Therapy Treatments May Increase Survival Rate in
Prostate Cancer Patients"
https://scitechdaily.com/hormone-therapy-treatments-may-
increase-survival-rate-in-prostate-cancer-patients/

"Popular 'Heart-Health' Supplements Found Ineffective at
Lowering Cholesterol"
2022
https://scitechdaily.com/popular-heart-health-supplements-
found-ineffective-at-lowering-cholesterol/

"100 Times Longer Than Previous Benchmarks—A Quantum
Breakthrough"
2022
https://scitechdaily.com/100-times-longer-than-previous-bench-
marks-a-quantum-breakthrough/

"10-Million-Years in the Making—Researchers Discover First-Ever
Documented Hybrid of Its Kind"
2022
https://scitechdaily.com/10-million-years-in-the-making-research-
ers-discover-first-ever-documented-hybrid-of-its-kind/

"Columbia Mass Murder Database Reveals Mass School Shootings
Are Not Caused by Mental Illness"
2022
https://scitechdaily.com/columbia-mass-murder-database-reveals-
mass-school-shootings-are-not-caused-by-mental-illness/

"Stanford Sleep Medicine Doctor Reveals How to Be a Morning Person"
2022
https://scitechdaily.com/stanford-sleep-medicine-doctor-reveals-
how-to-be-a-morning-person/

"The Testicular Hormones AMH, InhB, INSL3, and Testosterone
Can Be Independently Deficient in Older Men"
2017
https://academic.oup.com/biomedgerontology/
article-abstract/72/4/548/2630047

"Preserving Fertility in the Hypogonadal Patient: An Update"
2015
https://pubmed.ncbi.nlm.nih.gov/25337850/

Acknowledgments

To produce a state-of-the-art book on the breakthrough science of bioidentical hormone replacement therapy takes a village, a village of clinical expertise, experience, and a devotion to our now-brighter future in aging.

Special applause for the entire Advantage|Forbes Books creative team—especially to my writing coach, Bud Ramey, and my brilliant editorial manager, Lauren Steffes.

I acknowledge each of the key scientists, clinicians, and physicians who have contributed to *Restore* within the text. Our behind-the-scenes contributors have also been key to the overall success of this effort, and I express my deepest personal appreciation to these great colleagues:

- Tyler Brannon, esq., CEO, Optimal Bio

- Dr. Hamid Bakhteyar, Carolina Compounding

- Candi Brown, nurse practitioner

- Christian Davis, nurse practitioner

- Denise Verni, physician assistant

- Johnny Moody, nurse practitioner

- Mavis Jamal, physician assistant

- Shannon Converse, nurse practitioner

- Tanya Nix, DNP, nurse practitioner

- Kristen Malvesto, practice manager

- Jim Baker, principal, Optimal Bio

Endnotes

Preface

1   "A Journey of a Thousand Miles Begins with a Single Step," Literary Devices, accessed August 12, 2023 https://literarydevices. net/a-journey-of-a-thousand-miles-begins-with-a-single-step/.

2   Glen Llopis, "We Can't Prepare For Uncertainty Without Changing Our Ways," Forbes, August 2022, accessed September 21, 2023, https://www.forbes.com/sites/glennllopis/2022/08/13/we-cant-pre-pare-for-uncertainty-without-changing-our-ways/?sh=2937a1132f72.

3   "A Brief History of Human Longevity," Age Up, January 28, 2021, https://learn.age-up.com/blog/a-brief-history-of-human-longevity/.

4   Willie Drye, "The Fountain of Youth," National Geographic, accessed December 16, 2022, https://www.nationalgeographic.com/history/article/fountain-of-youth.

5   Drye, "The Fountain of Youth."

6   D. Benson, "Discover Restorative Medicine Conferences," Integrative Medicine (Encinitas), July 2022, https://www.ncbi.nlm.nih.gov/pmc/articles/PMC9380838/.

7   Randall Stock, "The Best of Sherlock Holmes," accessed July 5, 2023, http://www.bestofsherlock.com/top-10-sherlock-quotes. htm#impossible.

Introduction

8   "The Game Is Afoot," Literary Devices, accessed August 18m 2023, https://literarydevices.net/the-game-is-afoot/.

9   Cleveland Clinic, "What Are Bioidentical Hormones?," accessed January 19, 2023, https://my.clevelandclinic.org/health/articles/15660-bioidentical-hormones.

10   Sandee LaMotte, "Alzheimer's and HRT: Study Suggests Sweet
      Spot to Avoid Dementia," CNN, April 5, 2023, https://www.cnn.
      com/2023/04/03/health/alzheimers-hormone-replacement-therapy-
      wellness/index.html.

11   LaMotte, "Alzheimer's and HRT."

12   LaMotte, "Alzheimer's and HRT."

13   LaMotte, "Alzheimer's and HRT."

14   LaMotte, "Alzheimer's and HRT."

15   Scripts.com, "The Screenplay for *Indiana Jones and The Last Crusade*
      (1989)," accessed December 15, 2022, https://www.scripts.com/
      script/indiana_jones_and_the_last_crusade_480.

Chapter 1

16   Chrétien de Troyes, Ruth Harwood Cline (Translator), "*Perceval,
      or, The Story of the Grail, January 1, 1181*," accessed December
      19, 2022, https://www.goodreads.com/book/show/397023.
      Perceval_or_The_Story_of_the_Grail.

17   de Troyes, "Perceval."

18   Becky Little, "Knights Templar," National Geographic, May 12,
      2016, https://www.nationalgeographic.com/search?q=Knights%20
      Templar&location=srp&type=manual.

19   Little, "Knights Templar."

20   Little, "Knights Templar."

21   Glasonbury Abbey, "King Arthur and the Knights of the Round
      Table," accessed December 16, 2022, https://kingarthursknights.
      com/glastonbury-abbey/.

22   Glastonbury Abbey, "King Arthur."

23   King Arthur and the Knights of the Round Table, "Chalice Well
      Gardens in Glastonbury, England," accessed December 18, 2022,
      https://kingarthursknights.com/chalice-well-gardens/.

24   King Arthur, "Chalice Well Gardens."

25   "Medieval Histories," July 4, 2014, https://www.medieval.eu/
      holy-grail/.

26 "Medieval Histories."

27 "Found: 580-Year-Old Chinese Fountain of Youth Pill," UPI, June 25, 1982, https://www.upi.com/Archives/1982/06/25/Found-580-year-old-Chinese-fountain-of-youth-pill/9063393825600/.

28 Noah Charney, "Hitler's Hunt for the Holy Grail and the Ghent Altarpiece," Daily Beast, July 11, 2017, https://www.thedailybeast.com/hitlers-hunt-for-the-holy-grail-and-the-ghent-altarpiece.

29 Charney, "Hitler's Hunt for the Holy Grail."

30 "Medicinal Springs," Monticello.org, accessed December 16, 2022, https://www.monticello.org/research-education/thomas-jefferson-encyclopedia/medicinal-springs/.

31 Drye, "Fountain of Youth."

32 Sam Anderson, "My Search for the Fountain of Youth," The New York Times Magazine, October 24, 2014, https://www.nytimes.com/2014/10/26/magazine/my-search-for-the-fountain-of-youth.html.

33 Anderson, "My Search."

34 Anderson, "My Search."

35 "Fountain of Youth," Waymarking, accessed December 16, 2022, https://www.waymarking.com/waymarks/WMT2Z3_Fountain_of_Youth_Archeological_Park_St_Augustine_FL.

36 "Synopsis: Indiana Jones and the Last Crusade," Script Slug, accessed December 16, 2022, https://www.scriptslug.com/script/indiana-jones-and-the-last-crusade-1989.

37 Katharine Gammon, "It's time to rethink hormone therapy for women, says heart health scientist," Keck School of Medicine of USC, June 2021, accessed September 21, 2023, https://keck.usc.edu/its-time-to-rethink-hormone-therapy-for-women-says-heart-health-scientist.

Chapter 2

38 Katharine Gammon, "It's Time to Rethink Hormone Therapy for Women, Says Heart Health Scientist," USC Trojan, Spring 2021, https://news.usc.edu/trojan-family/benefits-hormone-replacement-therapy-women-estrogen-usc/.

39 Gammon, "It's Time to Rethink Hormone Therapy for Women."

40   Gammon, "It's Time to Rethink Hormone Therapy for Women."

41   Gammon, "It's Time to Rethink Hormone Therapy for Women."

42   Howard N. Hodis and Wendy J. Mack, "Menopausal Hormone Replacement Therapy and Reduction of All-Cause Mortality and Cardiovascular Disease: It's About Time and Timing," National Institutes of Health," May–June 2022, https://www.ncbi.nlm.nih.gov/pmc/articles/PMC9178928/#:~:text=showed%20that%20relative%20to%20placebo,)%20(24%2C25).

43   Hodis and Mack, "Menopausal Hormone Replacement Therapy."

44   Hodis and Mack, "Menopausal Hormone Replacement Therapy."

45   Hodis and Mack, "Menopausal Hormone Replacement Therapy."

46   Susan Dominus, "Women Have Been Misled About Menopause," New York Times, February 1, 2023, https://www.nytimes.com/2023/02/01/magazine/menopause-hot-flashes-hormone-therapy.html.

47   Dominus, "Women Have Been Misled."

48   J. W. Studd et al., "Issue 163," American Journal of Obstetrics and Gynecology, accessed March 18, 2023, https://www.sciencedirect.com/journal/american-journal-of-obstetrics-and-gynecology/vol/163/issue/6/part/P1.

49   Jay Campbell, "How to Optimize Your Testosterone for Lifelong Health and Happiness," *The Definitive Testosterone Replacement Therapy Manual*, 2015, 15.

50   Abraham Morgantaler, "Testosterone Therapy for Life," Life Extension Magazine, October 2021, https://www.lifeextension.com/magazine/2010/6/abraham-morgentaler-testosterone-therapy-for-life.

51   Morgantaler, "Testosterone Therapy for Life."

52   Morgantaler, "Testosterone Therapy for Life."

53   Morgantaler, "Testosterone Therapy for Life."

54   Gary S. Donovitz, "A Personal Perspective on Testosterone Therapy in Women—What We Know in 2022," Journal of Personalized Medicine, July 22, 2022, https://www.ncbi.nlm.nih.gov/pmc/articles/PMC9331845.

55   Donovitz, "A Personal Perspective."

56   Donovitz, "A Personal Perspective."

57   Donovitz, "A Personal Perspective."

58   Morgantaler, "Testosterone Therapy for Life."

59   Morgantaler, "Testosterone Therapy for Life."

60   Morgantaler, "Testosterone Therapy for Life."

61   Morgantaler, "Testosterone Therapy for Life."

62   Morgantaler, "Testosterone Therapy for Life."

63   Andrew Steele, *Ageless, The New Science of Getting Older Without Getting Old*, April 20, 2021, https://www.amazon.com/Ageless-Science-Getting-Older-Without/dp/059321479X.

64   Steele, *Ageless.*

65   Alex Moshakis, "Do We Have to Age?," The Guardian, January 3, 2021, https://www.theguardian.com/science/2021/jan/03/observer-magazine-do-we-have-to-age-biologist-andrew-steele.

66   Angelo Cagnacci and Martina Venier, "The Controversial History of Hormone Replacement Therapy," Medicina, September 2019, https://www.ncbi.nlm.nih.gov/pmc/articles/PMC6780820.

67   Cagnacci and Venier, "The Controversial History."

Chapter 3

68   Cleveland Clinic, "Hormones," accessed December 21, 2022, https://my.clevelandclinic.org/health/articles/22464-hormones.

69   Cleveland Clinic, "Hormones."

70   Cleveland Clinic, "Hormones."

71   "Writing Explained," accessed December 31, 2022, https://writing-explained.org/idiom-dictionary/cat-out-of-the-bag#:~:text=Let%20the%20Cat%20Out%20of%20the%20Bag%20Meaning,to%20stay%20hidden%20or%20unknown.

72   PETA, "Premarin: A Prescription for Cruelty," PETA, accessed December 27, 2022, https://www.peta.org/issues/animals-used-for-experimentation/premarin-hormone-replacement-therapy/.

73 Shelagh Niblock, "Continuous Improvement in Equine Ranching," CAA Horse Journal, accessed December 27, 2022, www.HorseJournals.com.

74 PETA, "Premarin."

75 Meryl Davids Landau, "The Wild History of Women's Hormone Therapy," Everyday Health, December 13, 2022, https://www.everydayhealth.com/womens-health/hormones/history-hormone-therapy/.

76 Landau, "The Wild History of Women's Hormone Therapy."

77 Landau, "The Wild History of Women's Hormone Therapy."

78 Gorazd Drevenšek et al., "Neurophysiological Repercussions of Anabolic Steroid Abuse: A Road to Neurodegenerative Disorders," *Sex Hormones in Neurodegenerative Processes and Diseases*, InTechOpen, London, May 2, 2018, https://www.intechopen.com/books/5994.

79 Drevenšek et al., "Neurophysiological Repercussions."

80 Drevenšek et al., "Neurophysiological Repercussions."

81 Landau, "The Wild History of Women's Hormone Therapy."

Chapter 4

82 Thomas Bangs Thorpe, *A Voice to America: The present Crisis in the United States*, (New York, 1855), 377, accessed December 19, 2022, https://www.amazon.com/Voice-America-Edward-Walker-ebook/dp/B07H2ZGN5T.

83 National Academies, *The Clinical Utility of Compounded Bioidentical Hormone Therapy, A Review of Safety, Effectiveness, and Use*, 5, accessed December 21, 2022, https://nap.nationalacademies.org/catalog/25791/the-clinical-utility-of-compounded-bioidentical-hormone-therapy-a-review.

84 National Academies, *The Clinical Utility*.

85 Diabetes.co.uk, "Men Experience an Abrupt Decrease in Testosterone Levels after Sugar Intake, Study Finds," Diabetes.co.uk, September 19, 2016, https://www.diabetes.co.uk/news/2016/sep/men-experience-an-abrupt-decrease-in-testosterone-levels-after-sugar-intake,-study-finds-99746064.html.

86   Healthline, "How Sleep Can Affect Your Hormone Levels," September 1, 2021, https://www.healthline.com/health/sleep/how-sleep-can-affect-your-hormone-levels.

87   Kavita Gandhi et al., "Exposure Risk and Environmental Impacts of Glyphosate: Highlights on the Toxicity of Herbicide Co-Formulants," Science Direct, August 2021, https://www.sciencedirect.com/science/article/pii/S2667010021001281.

88   CDC, "Thimerosal and Vaccines," Centers for Disease Control, accessed January 2, 2023, https://www.cdc.gov/vaccinesafety/concerns/thimerosal/index.html.

89   EPA, "Minamata Convention on Mercury," Environmental Protection Agency, accessed January 3, 2023, https://www.epa.gov/international-cooperation/minamata-convention-mercury.

90   Andrew McCullough, "A Review of Testosterone Pellets in the Treatment of Hypogonadism," National Institutes of Health, October 3, 2014, https://www.ncbi.nlm.nih.gov/pmc/articles/PMC4431706/.

91   Frédéric Bastiat, *The Law*, June 1850, v, accessed December 17, 2022, http://bastiat.org/en/the_law.html.

92   Robert Malone, "Health, Aging and Hormonal Balance," Who Is Robert Malone?, March 24, 2022, https://rwmalonemd.substack.com/p/health-aging-and-hormonal-balance.

93   Malone, "Health, Aging and Hormonal Balance."

94   J. R. Fishman et al., "Bioidentical Hormones, Menopausal Women, and the Lure of the 'Natural' in US Anti-Aging Medicine," Journal of Science and Medicine, May 2015, https://www.ncbi.nlm.nih.gov/pmc/articles/PMC4400226/.

95   Bastiat, *The Law*.

96   Bastiat, *The Law*.

97   Bastiat, *The Law*.

98   Bastiat, *The Law*.

99   Bastiat, *The Law*.

100 Despina G. Contopoulos-Ioannidis et al., "Life Cycle of Translational Research," PolicyForum, September 5, 2008.

101 Despina G. Contopoulos-Ioannidis et al., "Life Cycle of Translational Research."

102 Despina G. Contopoulos-Ioannidis et al., "Life Cycle of Translational Research."

103 Bastiat, *The Law.*

104 "About the Books," Alan Alda, accessed January 15, 2023, http://www.alanalda.com/alan_alda_about_the_books.php.

105 Alison Beard, "Life's Work: An Interview with Alan Alda," Harvard Business Review, July–August 2017, https://hbr.org/2017/07/alan-alda.

106 Beard, "Life's Work."

107 "Male Fertility Is Declining—Studies Show That Environmental Toxins Could Be a Reason," The Conversation, July 30, 2021, https://theconversation.com/male-fertility-is-declining-studies-show-that-environmental-toxins-could-be-a-reason-163795.

108 "Evidence for Decreasing Quality of Semen during Past 50 years," British Medical Journal, September 12, 1992, https://www.bmj.com/content/305/6854/609.

109 Cleveland Clinic, "Low Testosterone, Male Hypogonadism," accessed February 26, 2023, https://my.clevelandclinic.org/health/diseases/15603-low-testosterone-male-hypogonadism.

110 Clevalend Clinic, "Low Testosterone."

111 Cleveland Clinic, "Lifestyle Choices Are Often a Contributing Factor for Low-T," September 20, 2022, https://health.clevelandclinic.org/declining-testosterone-levels/#:~:text=It's%20normal%20for%20testosterone%20levels,same%20age%20in%20different%20years.

112 T.G. Travison et al., "A Population-Level Decline in Serum Testosterone Levels in American Men," Journal of Clinical Endocrinology and Metabolism, January 2007, https://pubmed.ncbi.nlm.nih.gov/17062768/.

113 Travison et al., "A Population-Level Decline."

114 Travison et al., "A Population-Level Decline."

115 CDC, "Strengthening Clinicl Labs," Centers for Disease Control, accessed January 15, 2023, https://www.cdc.gov/csels/dls/strengthening-clinical-labs.html.

116 ClinLab Navigator, "Aging Effect on Laboratory Values," accessed January 14, 2023, http://www.clinlabnavigator.com/aging-effect-on-laboratory-values.html.

117 LabCorp, "Q&A: Testosterone," accessed August 19, 2023, https://www.labcorp.com/assets/11476.

118 D. J. Topliss, "What Happens When Laboratory Reference Ranges Change," CMAJ, May 4, 2020, https://www.ncbi.nlm.nih.gov/pmc/articles/PMC7207180/.

119 Topliss, "What Happens."

120 Topliss, "What Happens."

121 Susan R. Davis et al., "Global Consensus Position Statement on the Use of Testosterone Therapy for Women," *The Journal of Clinical Endocrinology & Metabolism* 104, no. 10 (October 2019), https://doi.org/10.1210/jc.2019-01603.

122 Howard Markel, "The Awful Work of the Real Doctors Who Inspired *M*A*S*H*," PBS, February 28, 2019, https://www.pbs.org/newshour/health/the-awful-work-of-the-real-doctors-who-inspired-mash.

123 Howard Fishman, "What *M*A*S*H* Taught Us," The New Yorker, July 24, 2018, https://www.newyorker.com/culture/culture-desk/what-mash-taught-us.

The Miracle of Our Hormones

124 Susanne Hiller-Sturmhöfel and Andrzej Bartke, "The Endocrine System: An Overview," US National Institutes of Health, National Cancer Institute, accessed April 24, 2023, https://www.ncbi.nlm.nih.gov/pmc/articles/PMC6761896/.

125 Maggie Armstrong et al., "Physiology, Thyroid Function," National Library of Medicine, March 13, 2023, https://www.ncbi.nlm.nih.gov/books/NBK537039/#:~:text=The%20thyroid%20produces%20approximately%2090,%2C%20or%20triiodothyronine%20(T3).

Chapter 5

126 Suzanne Somers, "I Have My …," Brainy Quote, accessed February 27, 2023 https://www.brainyquote.com/quotes/suzanne_somers_281170?src=t_hormones.

127 Somers, "I Have My …"

128 Susan M. Sawyer et al., "Child and Adolescent Health," The Lancet, January 17, 2018, https://www.thelancet.com/journals/lanchi/article/PIIS2352-4642%2818%2930022-1/fulltext.

129 US History, "The Invention of the Teenager," accessed January 15, 2023, https://www.ushistory.org/us/46c.asp.

130 Interesting Literature, "Ugly Duckling," accessed January 9, 2023, https://interestingliterature.com/2020/05/ugly-duckling-fairy-tale-andersen-summary-analysis.

131 Suva Biturogoiwasa, "My Village, My World: Everyday Life in Nadoria, Fiji," Institute of Pacific Studies, The University of the South Pacific, October 18, 2019, https://www.actionaid.org.uk/blog/news/2019/10/18/how-do-people-around-the-world-celebrate-periods#footnote2_f4oul9j.

132 Carol A. Markstrom, "Empowerment of North American Indian Girls: Ritual Expressions at Puberty," Actionaid.org. October 18, 2019, https://www.actionaid.org.uk/blog/news/2019/10/18/how-do-people-around-the-world-celebrate-periods#footnote2_f4oul9j.

133 Mayo Clinic, "Depression in Women: Understanding the Gender Gap," Mayo Clinic, accessed February 27, 2023, https://www.mayoclinic.org/diseases-conditions/depression/in-depth/depression/art-20047725#:~:text=Women%20are%20nearly%20twice%20as,alone%20don't%20cause%20depression.

134 Mayo Cinic, "Depression in Women."

135 Society for Endocrinology, "You and Your Hormones," accessed March 27, 2023, https://www.yourhormones.info/hormones/luteinising-hormone/.

136 Society for Endocrinology, "You and Your Hormones."

137 American Society for Reproductive Medicine, "Age and Fertility," accessed January 12, 2023, https://www.reproductivefacts.org/

news-and-publications/patient-fact-sheets-and-booklets/documents/
fact-sheets-and-info-booklets/age-and-fertility/.

138 American Society for Reproductive Medicine, "Age and Fertility,"

139 Society for Endocrinology, "You and Your Hormones."

140 Johns Hopkins Medicine, "Low Levels of Anxiety Hormone Linked
to Postpartum Depression," accessed January 12, 2023, https://
www.hopkinsmedicine.org/news/media/releases/low_levels_of_anti_
anxiety_hormone_linked_to_postpartum_depression.

141 Natural Womanhood, "Overcome Postpartum Depression with Bioidentical Progeterone," accessed
January 12, 2023, https://naturalwomanhood.org/
overcome-postpartum-depression-with-bioidentical-progesterone/.

142 Natural Womanhood, "Overcome Postpartum Depression."

143 Suzanne Somers, *Ageless: The Naked Truth About Bioidentical Hormones*, December 31, 2007, https://www.amazon.com/
Ageless-Naked-Truth-Bioidentical-Hormones/dp/0307237257.

144 Harvard Health, "Hot Flashes and Heart Health," Harvard Women's
Health, accessed January 12, 2023, https://www.health.harvard.
edu/womens-health/hot-flashes-and-heart-health#:~:text=This%20
symptom%20is%20common%20in,40)%20and%20certain%20
pregnancy%20complications.

145 Harvard Health, "Hot Flashes and Heart Health."

146 Harvard Health, "Hot Flashes and Heart Health."

147 Gorazd Drevenšek, *Sex Hormones in Neurodegenerative Processes and
Diseases*, InTechOpen, London, May 2, 2018, ix–xii, https://www.
intechopen.com/books/5994.

148 Drevenšek, *Sex Hormones.*

149 Drevenšek, *Sex Hormones.*

150 Drevenšek, *Sex Hormones.*

151 Drevenšek, *Sex Hormones.*

152 Drevenšek, *Sex Hormones.*

153 Drevenšek, *Sex Hormones.*

154 Drevenšek, *Sex Hormones.*

155 Julie A. Elder et al., "Menopause," Cleveland Clinic, February 2016, https://www.clevelandclinicmeded.com/medicalpubs/diseasemanagement/womens-health/menopause/#:~:text=Estrone%20(E1)%20is%20the%20dominant,of%20androstenedione%20in%20adipose%20tissue.

156 CDC, "Women," Centers for Disease Control, accessed January 13, 2023, https://www.cdc.gov/women/lcod/2017/all-races-origins/index.htm.

157 CDC, "Women."

158 CDC, "Women."

159 Laurie Toich, "Breast Cancer Rates Vary Substantially in the US, Japan," Pharmacy Times, August 2, 2017, https://www.pharmacytimes.com/view/breast-cancer-rates-vary-substantially-in-the-us-japan.

160 Laurie Toich, "Breast Cancer Rates."

161 "HRT and Breast Cancer Risk," British Medical Journal, accessed March 2, 2023, https://www.bmj.com/content/367/bmj.l5928/rr-3.

162 Agnès Fournier et al., "Unequal Risks for Breast Cancer Associated with Different Hormone Replacement Therapies: Results from the E3N Cohort Study," National Library of Medicine, January 2008, https://www.ncbi.nlm.nih.gov/pmc/articles/PMC2211383/.

163 Fournier et al., "Unequal Risks for Breast Cancer."

164 Maggie Fox, "One in 6 Americans Take Antidepressants, Other Psychiatric Drugs: Study," NBC News, December 12, 2016, https://www.nbcnews.com/health/health-news/one-6-americans-take-antidepressants-other-psychiatric-drugs-NBCn695141.

165 Johns Hopkins Medicine, "What Is Perimenopause?," accessed January 13, 2023, https://www.hopkinsmedicine.org/health/conditions-and-diseases/perimenopause.

166 Johns Hopkins Medicine, "What Is Perimenopause?."

167 Julia Prague, "Menopause: Life After Reproduction: The Slow Moon Climbs: The Science, History, and Meaning of Menopause," Nature, October 1, 2019, https://www.nature.com/articles/d41586-019-02940-7.

168 Lekha Adik Pathak et al., "Coronary Artery Disease in Women," Indian Heart Journal, July–August 2017, http://www.ncbi.nlm.nih.gov/pmc/articles/PMC5560902/.

169 Endocrine Society, "Menopause and Bone Loss," January 24, 2022, https://www.endocrine.org/patient-engagement/endocrine-library/menopause-and-bone-loss.

170 Endocrine Society, "Menopause and Bone Loss."

171 *Journal of the North American Menopause Association*, May 2022, https://www.menopause.org/docs/default-source/professional/nams-2022-hormone-therapy-position-statement.pdf.

172 Rush, "Hormones as You Age," accessed January 13, 2023, https://www.rush.edu/news/hormones-you-age.

173 Carol Tavris and Avrum Bluming, *Estrogen Matters: Why Taking Hormones in Menopause Can Improve Women's Well-Being and Lengthen Their Lives—Without Raising the Risk of Breast Cancer*, September 4, 2018, https://www.amazon.com/Estrogen-Matters-Hormones-Menopause-Well-Being-ebook/dp/B078W61N8Z/ref=sr_1_1?crid=3DWBISN7D8079&keywords=Estrogen+Matters&qid=1673016953&s=books&sprefix=estrogen+matters%2Cstripbooks%2C58&sr=1-1.

174 Johns Hopkins Medicine, "Health," accessed March 5, 2023, https://www.hopkinsmedicine.org/health/conditions-and-diseases/osteoporosis.

175 Marco Gambacciani and Marco Levancin, "Hormone Replacement Therapy and the Prevention of Postmenopausal Osteoporosis," National Library of Medicine, *Menopause Review*, September 9, 2014, https://www.ncbi.nlm.nih.gov/pmc/articles/PMC4520366/.

176 Jean Pincott, "Menopause Predisposes a Fifth of Women to Alzheimer's," Scientific American, May 1, 2020, https://www.scientificamerican.com/article/menopause-predisposes-a-fifth-of-women-to-alzheimers/.

177 Jean Pincott, "Menopause Predisposes a Fifth of Women."

178 Jean Pincott, "Menopause Predisposes a Fifth of Women."

Chapter 6

179 M. Westwood and J. Pinzon, "Adolescent Male Health," Pediatric Child Health, January 2008, https://www.ncbi.nlm.nih.gov/pmc/articles/PMC2528816/.

180 Kariega Game Reserve, "Lion Cubs: 12 Interesting Facts," accessed January 22, 2023, https://www.kariega.co.za/blog/lion-cubs-12-interestingfacts#:~:text=Lion%20cubs%20are%20quick%20devel-opers, for%20up%20to%20two%20months.

181 Kariega Game Reserve, "Lion Cubs: 12 Interesting Facts."

182 Johns Hopkins Medicine, "Puberty: Adolescent Male," accessed January 22, 2023, https://www.hopkinsmedicine.org/health/wellness-and-prevention/puberty-adolescent-male#:~:text=Hair%20will%20start%20to%20grow,in%20oily%20skin%20and%20sweating.

183 The Positive Mom, "The Most Powerful Life Lessons From 'The Lion King,'" accessed January 22, 2023, https://www.thepositivemom.com/life-lessons-from-the-lion-king.

184 Mayo Clinic, "Metabolic Syndrome," accessed January 22, 2023, https://www.mayoclinic.org/diseases-conditions/metabolic-syndrome/symptoms-causes/syc-20351916#:~:text=Metabolic%20syndrome%20is%20a%20cluster,abnormal%20cholesterol%20or%20triglyceride%20levels.

185 "Most Heart Attack Patients' Cholesterol Levels Did Not Indicate Cardiac Risk," Science Daily, January 13, 2009, https://www.science-daily.com/releases/2009/01/090112130653.htm.

186 Elizabeth Millard, "What to Know if Your Doctor Put You on Statins to Lower Cholesterol," Time, January 25, 2023, accessed March 17, 2023.

187 Elizabeth Millard, "What to Know."

188 Elizabeth Millard, "What to Know."

189 David Diamond, "Statin Use Not Justified for Healthy People with High Cholesterol," University of South Florida Newsroom, September 19, 2022, https://www.usf.edu/news/2022/usf-professor-

statin-use-not-justified-for-healthy-people-with-high-cholesterol.
aspx.

190 David Diamond, "Statin Use Not Justified."

191 David Diamond, "Statin Use Not Justified."

192 David M. Diamond et al., "Statin Therapy Is Not Warranted for
a Person with High LDL-Cholesterol on a Low-Carbohydrate
Diet," October 2022, https://journals.lww.com/co-endocrinology/
Fulltext/2022/10000/Statin_therapy_is_not_warranted_for_a_
person_with.14.aspx.

193 David M. Diamond et al., "Statin Therapy Is Not Warranted."

194 Health Matters, "Lipoprotein Particles and Apolipoproteins: LDL
Particle Number," accessed August 22, 2023, https://healthmatters.
io/understand-blood-test-results/ldl-particle-number.

195 Health Matters, "Lipoprotein Particles and Apolipoproteins."

196 Health Matters, "Lipoprotein Particles and Apolipoproteins."

197 Women's Health Network, "Endocrine disruptors—The Hormonal
Effects of Everyday Toxins," accessed March 3, 2023, https://www.
womenshealthnetwork.com/detoxification/endocrine-disruptors/.

198 Medanta, "Patient Education: Signs You Are Experiencing Hormone Imbalance," accessed January 22, 2023,
https://www.medanta.org/patient-education-blog/
signs-youre-experiencing-a-hormone-imbalance-for-men/.

199 Ann Kearns, "Adrenal Fatigue: What Causes It?," Mayo Clinic,
accessed March 3, 2023, https://www.mayoclinic.org/diseases-
conditions/addisons-disease/expert-answers/adrenal-fatigue/
faq-20057906.

200 Kearns, "Adrenal Fatigue."

201 Cleveland Clinic, "Thyroid Disease," accessed January 25, 2023,
https://my.clevelandclinic.org/health/diseases/8541-thyroid-disease.

202 Mayo Clinic, "Hyperthyroidism," accessed January 25, 2023,
https://www.mayoclinic.org/diseases-conditions/hyperthyroidism/
symptoms-causes/syc-20373659#:~:text=Hyperthyroidism%20
happens%20when%20the%20thyroid,and%20rapid%20or%20
irregular%20heartbeat.

203   Journal of the American Medical Association, "Low Serum
      Testosterone Mortality in Male Veterans," JAMA, August 14,
      2006, https://jamanetwork.com/journals/jamainternalmedi-
      cine/fullarticle/410768#:~:text=In%20an%20unadjusted%20
      model%2C%20low,men%20with%20normal%20testosterone%20
      levels.

204   Journal of the American Medical Association, "Low Serum Testoster-
      one Mortality."

205   Journal of the American Medical Association, "Low Serum Testoster-
      one Mortality."

206   Journal of the American Medical Association, "Low Serum Testoster-
      one Mortality."

207   Mayo Clinic, "Sexual Health: Tips for Older Men," accessed January
      26, 2023, https://www.mayoclinic.org/healthy-lifestyle/sexual-health/
      in-depth/senior-sex/art-20046465.

208   Genius Lyrics, "When I'm 64," accessed July 13, 2023, https://
      genius.com/The-beatles-when-im-sixty-four-lyrics.

209   Atiyah Tidd-Johnson et al., "Prostate Cancer Screening:
      Continued Controversies and Novel Biomarker Advance-
      ments," Current Urology, December 2022, https://
      journals.lww.com/cur/Fulltext/2022/12000/
      Prostate_cancer_screening__Continued_controversies.2.aspx.

210   Tidd-Johnson et al., "Prostate Cancer Screening."

211   Natalie C. Ward et al., "Statin Toxicity, Mechanistic Insights,
      and Clinical Implications," Circulation Research, accessed
      January 25, 2023, https://www.ahajournals.org/doi/full/10.1161/
      CIRCRESAHA.118.312782.

212   Elizabeth Rosenthal, An American Sickness: How Healthcare Became
      Big Business and How You Can Take It Back, April 11, 2017, https://
      www.amazon.com/American-Sickness-Healthcare-Became-Business-
      ebook/dp/B01IOHQ9LO/ref=sr_1_1?ie=UTF8&qid=1497474913
      &sr=8-1&keywords=an+american+sickness.

213   Mayo Clinic, "Male Menopause, Myth or Reality?," accessed July
      13, 2023, https://www.mayoclinic.org/healthy-lifestyle/mens-health/
      in-depth/male-menopause/art-20048056.

214 Lawlinguists, "English Translation of 'The Circle of Life," accessed March 3, 2023, https://lawlinguists.com/English-translation-circle-life/.

Chapter 7

215 Washburn Hopkins, "Fountain of Youth," *Journal of the American Oriental Society* 26, 1905, accessed February 4, 2023, https://www.jstor.org/stable/pdf/592875.pdf.

216 Hopkins, "Fountain of Youth."

217 Hopkins, "Fountain of Youth."

218 Peter Attia, *Outlive: The Science and Art of Longevity* (New York City: Random House, 2023), 81–82.

219 Attia, *Outlive*.

220 *Health Encyclopedia*, "Total Testosterone," accessed February 8, 2023, https://www.urmc.rochester.edu/encyclopedia/content.aspx?contenttypeid=167&contentid=testosterone_total.

221 Mayo Clinic, "Endocrinology Catalog: Testosterone, Total and Bio-available, Serum," accessed February 8, 2023, https://endocrinology.testcatalog.org/show/TTBS.

222 Labcorp, "Testosterone Total," accessed February 8, 2023 https://www.labcorp.com/tests/004226/testosterone-total.

223 Quest Diagnostics, "Testosterone Total, MS," accessed February 8, 2023, https://testdirectory.questdiagnostics.com/test/test-detail/15983/testosterone-total-ms?cc=MASTER.

224 Bioreference Laboratories, "Client Update," accessed February 8, 2023, https://www.bioreference.com/wp-content/uploads/2019/10/October-Client-Update.pdf.

225 Charu Mahajan et al., "Endocrine Dysfunction after Traumatic Brain Injury: An Ignored Clinical Syndrome?," Neuro Critical Care Society, February 2003, https://doi.org/10.1007/s12028-022-01672-3.

226 Mahajan et al., "Endocrine Dysfunction after Traumatic Brain Injury."

227 W. Heaton, "What Role Does Progesterone Play in Thyroid Function?," Palmetto Bella Magazine, October

8, 2016, https://palmettobella.com/2016/10/08/
role-progesterone-play-thyroid-function/.

228 Noor Asi et al., "Progesterone vs. Synthetic Progestins and the Risk
of Breast Cancer: A Systematic Review and Meta-Analysis," July
2016, https://pubmed.ncbi.nlm.nih.gov/27456847.

229 Asi et al., "Progesterone vs. Synthetic Progestins."

230 E. Diamanti-Kandarakis et al., "Endocrine-Disrupting Chemicals:
An Endocrine Society Scientific Statement," Endocrine Review, July
2009, https://pubmed.ncbi.nlm.nih.gov/19502515/.

231 Diamanti-Kandarakis et al., "Endocrine-Disrupting Chemicals."

232 Cleveland Clinic, "Thyroid Disease," accessed March 8, 2023,
https://my.clevelandclinic.org/health/diseases/8541-thyroid-disease.

233 Hopkins Medicine, "Thyroid Disorders in Women," accessed
March 8, 2023, https://www.hopkinsmedicine.org/health/
conditions-and-diseases/thyroid-disorders-in-women.

234 Hopkins Medicine, "Thyroid Disorders in Women."

235 Cleveland Clinic, "Thyroid Disease."

236 Encyclopaedia.com, "Halogens," accessed July 13, 2023, https://
www.encyclopedia.com/science-and-technology/chemistry/
compounds-and-elements/halogen-elements.

237 National Institutes of Health, "Iodine, Fact Sheet for Health Professionals," NIH Office of Dietary Supplements, accessed March 11,
2023, https://ods.od.nih.gov/factsheets/Iodine-HealthProfessional/.

238 National Institutes of Health, "Iodine."

239 National Institutes of Health, "Iodine."

240 National Institutes of Health, "Iodine."

241 Carmen Aceves et al., "The Extrathyronine Actions of Iodine as Anti-
oxidant, Apoptotic, and Differentiation Factor in Various Tissues,"
Thyroid, August 2013, https://www.ncbi.nlm.nih.gov/pmc/articles/
PMC3752513/.

242 Aceves et al., "The Extrathyronine Actions of Iodine."

243 James A. Pittman et al., "Changing Normal Values for Thyroidal
Radioiodine Uptake," New England Journal of Medicine,

June 26, 1969, https://www.nejm.org/doi/full/10.1056/
NEJM196906262802602.

244 CDC, Iodine Level, Centers for Disease Control, National Center
for Health Statistics, accessed March 8, 2023, https://www.cdc.gov/
nchs/data/hestat/iodine.htm.

245 David Brownstein, "Busting the Iodine Myths," Forum Health,
January 10, 2017, https://www.power2practice.com/article/
busting-the-iodine-myths/.

246 Jarred Younger et al., "The Use of Low-Dose Naltrexone (LDN) as
a Novel Anti-Inflammatory Treatment for Chronic Pain," Clinical
Rheumatology, February 15, 2014, https://www.ncbi.nlm.nih.gov/
pmc/articles/PMC3962576/.

247 NIH, "Fact Sheet for Vitamin D for Health Professionals,"
National Institutes of Health, Office of Dietary Supplements,
accessed March 11, 2023, https://ods.od.nih.gov/factsheets/
VitaminD-HealthProfessional/.

248 Mercola, "Vitamin D Resource Page," accessed March 11, 2023,
https://www.mercola.com/article/vitamin-d-resources.htm.

249 National Cancer Institute, "Vitamin D Supplements Don't
Reduce Cancer Incidence, Trial Shows," December 13, 2018,
https://www.cancer.gov/news-events/cancer-currents-blog/2018/
vitamin-d-supplement-cancer-prevention.

250 National Cancer Institute, "Vitamin D Supplements."

251 NIH, "Fact Sheet for Vitamin D."

252 NIH, "Fact Sheet for Vitamin D."

253 NIH, "Fact Sheet for Vitamin D."

254 Kate Rhéaume, "Vitamin K2 and the Calcium Paradox: How
a Little-Known Vitamin Could Save Your Life," Doctorkatend.
com, accessed March 11, 2023, https://www.doctorkatend.com/
vitamin-k2-and-the-calcium-paradox/.

255 Rhéaume, "Vitamin K2 and the Calcium Paradox."

256 Rhéaume, "Vitamin K2 and the Calcium Paradox."

257 A. K. Heath et al., "Vitamin D Status and Mortality: A Systematic
Review of Observational Studies," International Journal of Environ-

mental Research and Public Health, January 2019, https://www.ncbi. nlm.nih.gov/pmc/articles/PMC6388383/.

258 Mohit Khera, "Adult-Onset Hypogonadism," Mayo Clinic, July 2016, http://dx.doi.org/10.1016/j.mayocp.2016.04.022.

259 Khera, "Adult-Onset Hypogonadism."

260 Khera, "Adult-Onset Hypogonadism."

261 American Cancer Society, "Key Statistics for Prostate Cancer," accessed July 14, 2023, https://www.cancer.org/cancer/types/ prostate-cancer/about/key-statistics.html#:~:text=About%201%20 man%20in%208,rare%20in%20men%20under%2040.

262 American Cancer Society, "Key Statistics for Prostate Cancer."

263 Richard M. Hoffman, "Screening for Prostate Cancer," UpToDate, February 2023, https://www.uptodate.com/contents/ screening-for-prostate-cancer#H25.

264 Hoffman, "Screening for Prostate Cancer."

265 Weill Cornell Medicine, "Less Prostate Cancer Screening Reduces Overdiagnosis but May Miss Aggressive Cases," April 22, 2022, https://news.weill.cornell.edu/news/2022/04/less-prostate-cancer-screening-reduces-overdiagnosis-but-may-miss-aggressive-cases.

266 Weill Cornell Medicine, "Less Prostate Cancer Screening."

267 US Preventive Services Task Force, "Prostate Cancer Screening," accessed July 14, 2023, https://www.uspreventiveservicestaskforce. org/uspstf/recommendation/prostate-cancer-screening.

268 Weill Cornell Medicine, "Less Prostate Cancer Screening."

269 Weill Cornell Medicine, "Less Prostate Cancer Screening."

270 Weill Cornell Medicine, "Less Prostate Cancer Screening."

271 Weill Cornell Medicine, "Less Prostate Cancer Screening."

272 Mayo Clinic, "Fundamental Concepts Regarding Testosterone Deficiency and Treatment, International Expert Consensus Resolutions," Mayo Clinic Proceedings accessed February 8, 2023, https://www. mayoclinicproceedings.org/article/S0025-6196(16)30115-X/fulltext.

273 Mayo Clinic, "Fundamental Concepts Regarding Testosterone Deficiency."

274 Mayo Clinic, "Fundamental Concepts Regarding Testosterone Deficiency."

275 CDC, "National Diabetes Statistics Report," reviewed June 2022, accessed September 21, 2023, https://www.cdc.gov/diabetes/data/statistics-report/index.html.

Chapter 8

276 Kevin D. Hall and Scott Kahan, "Maintenance of Lost Weight and Long-Term Management of Obesity," National Library of Medicine, January 2018, https://www.ncbi.nlm.nih.gov/pmc/articles/PMC5764193/.

277 Hall and Kahan, "Maintenance of Lost Weight."

278 Medical News Today, "What to Know about Peptides for Health," March 30, 2023, https://www.medicalnewstoday.com/articles/326701#about.

279 Medical News Today, "What to Know about Peptides."

280 National Institutes of Health, "Steroids and Other Appearance and Performance Enhancing Drugs (APEDs) Research Report: Are Anabolic Steroids Addictive?," National Institute on Drug Abuse, February 2018, https://nida.nih.gov/publications/research-reports/steroids-other-appearance-performance-enhancing-drugs-apeds/are-anabolic-steroids-addictive.

281 National Institutes of Health, "Steroids and Other …"

282 William Seeds, *The Peptide Protocols*, accessed March 17, 2023, https://www.amazon.com/Peptide-Protocols-William-Seeds-MD/dp/0578624354?asin=B08LZLYCXL&revisionId=ff7bab5c&format=1&depth=1Growth, 2020.

283 Seeds, *The Peptide Protocols*.

284 Seeds, *The Peptide Protocols*.

285 Seeds, *The Peptide Protocols*.

286 Cristina Martínez-Villaluenga and Blanca Hernández-Ledesma, "Peptides for Health Benefits 2020," International Journal of Molecular Science, June 16, 2020, https://www.ncbi.nlm.nih.gov/pmc/articles/PMC9223426/.

287 Martínez-Villaluenga and Hernández-Ledesma, "Peptides."

288 Lei Wang et al., "Therapeutic Peptides: Current Applications and Future Directions," Nature, February 2022, https://www.nature.com/articles/s41392-022-00904-4.

289 Wang et al., "Therapeutic Peptides."

290 Wang et al., "Therapeutic Peptides."

291 The Food Historian, "The Basic Seven," accessed August 19, 2023, https://www.thefoodhistorian.com/blog/world-war-wednesdays-the-basic-seven.

292 Randall Fitzgerald, *The Hundred-Year Lie: How Food and Medicine Are Destroying Your Health* (New York, 2006), 13.

293 Dietary Goals for the United States, accessed August 19, 2023, https://zerodisease.com/archive/Dietary_Goals_For_The_United_States.pdf.

294 Ecosystems United, "A History of the Development of the Food Pyramid and Dietary Guidelines in the United States," accessed January 23, 2023, https://ecosystemsunited.com/2014/08/13/the-food-pyramid-a-brief-history/.

295 Ecosystems United, "A History of the Development of the Food Pyramid."

296 P. Grasgruber et al., "Food Consumption and the Actual Statistics of Cardiovascular Diseases: An Epidemiological Comparison of 42 European Countries," Food & Nutrition Research, accessed March 31, 2023, https://pubmed.ncbi.nlm.nih.gov/27680091/.

297 M. Dehghan, et al., "Associations of Fats and Carbohydrate Intake with Cardiovascular Disease and Mortality in 18 Countries from Five Continents (PURE): A Prospective Cohort Study," The Lancet, November 4, 2017, https://pubmed.ncbi.nlm.nih.gov/28864332/.

298 Joseph E. Scherger, "The Diabetes Code," Family Medicine, May 2019, https://journals.stfm.org/familymedicine/2019/march/br-mar19-scherger.

299 Scherger, "The Diabetes Code."

300 Scherger, "The Diabetes Code."

301 Scherger, "The Diabetes Code."

302 Scherger, "The Diabetes Code."

303 Merrill Matschke, "Erectile Dysfunction as an Indicator of Cardio-vascular Disease & Early Death," Levels: Metabolic Insights, January 24, 2023, https://www.levelshealth.com/blog/erectile-dysfunction-as-an-indicator-of-cardiovascular-disease-early-death.

304 Matschke, "Erectile Dysfunction."

305 Matschke, "Erectile Dysfunction."

306 Matschke, "Erectile Dysfunction."

307 Matschke, "Erectile Dysfunction."

308 Matschke, "Erectile Dysfunction."

309 Matschke, "Erectile Dysfunction."

310 Matschke, "Erectile Dysfunction."

311 Barbara Branning, "UB Diabetes Expert's Research Shows Testoster-one Therapy Can Lead to Remission in Men with Type 2 Diabetes," University of Buffalo News Center, July 29, 2020, https://www.buffalo.edu/news/releases/2020/07/018.html.

312 Branning, "UB Diabetes Expert's Research."

313 Branning, "UB Diabetes Expert's Research."

314 Joseph M. Mercola, "Ten Common Nutrient Deficiencies," Take Control, May 17, 2022, https://takecontrol.substack.com/p/10-common-nutrient-deficiencies.

315 Mercola, "Ten Common Nutrient Deficiencies."

316 Mercola, "Ten Common Nutrient Deficiencies."

317 Joseph Mercola, "Time-Restricted Eating—A Powerful Way to Prevent Dementia," LewRockwell.com, March 30, 2020, https://www.lewrockwell.com/2020/03/joseph-mercola/time-restricted-eating-a-powerful-way-to-prevent-dementia/.

318 Yi Yang and Lihui Zhang, "The Effects of Caloric Restriction and Its Mimetics in Alzheimer's Disease through Autophagy Pathways," Food Function, February 26, 2020, https://pubmed.ncbi.nlm.nih.gov/32068753/.

319 Yang and Zhang, "The Effects of Caloric Restriction."

320 Gina Kolata and Francesca Paris, "The Medicine Is a Miracle, but Only if You Can Afford It," New York Times, February 7, 2023, https://www.nytimes.com/2023/02/07/health/medicine-insurance-payments.html.

321 Benjamin N. Rome et al., "Trends in Prescription Drug Launch Prices, 2008–2021," JAMA Network, June 7, 2022, https://jamanetwork.com/journals/jama/article-abstract/2792986.

322 Rome et al., "Trends in Prescription Drug Launch Prices."

323 Rome et al., "Trends in Prescription Drug Launch Prices."

324 American Academy of Dermatology, "Do You Have Hair Loss or Hair Shedding?," AAD.org, accessed July 14, 2023, https://www.aad.org/public/diseases/hair-loss/insider/shedding.

325 J. Abram McBride and Robert M. Coward, "Recovery of Spermatogenesis Following Testosterone Replacement Therapy or Anabolic-Androgenic Steroid Use," National Library of Medicine, May–June 2016, https://www.ncbi.nlm.nih.gov/pmc/articles/PMC4854084/.

Chapter 9

326 CDC, "Deaths from Older Adult Falls," Centers for Disease Control, accessed March 19, 2023, https://www.cdc.gov/falls/data/fall-deaths.html#:~:text=Falls%20are%20the%20leading%20cause,fall%20death%20rate%20is%20increasing.&text=The%20age%2Dadjusted%20fall%20death%20rate%20increased%20by%2041%25%20from,100%2C000%20older%20adults%20in%202021.

327 The University of Rochester, "Lays of the Round Table and Other Lyric Romances," The Camelot Project, accessed March 19, 2023, https://d.lib.rochester.edu/camelot/text/rhys-quest-of-the-grail-on-the-eve.

328 VCU News, "For Older Adults, 'Hope' May Be a Key Piece for Improving Health, Psychological and Social Well-Being," Virginia Commonwealth University, February 14, 2020, https://www.news.vcu.edu/article/For_older_adults_hope_may_be_a_key_piece_for_improving_health.

329 VCU News, "For Older Adults."

330 VCU News, "For Older Adults."

331 VCU News, "For Older Adults."

332 VCU News, "For Older Adults."

333 VCU News, "For Older Adults."

334 VCU News, "For Older Adults."

335 VCU News, "For Older Adults."

336 VCU News, "For Older Adults."

337 Endocrine Society, "New Defined Reference Range Can Help Limit Misdiagnoses and Unnecessary Treatments," Journal of Clinical Endocrinology & Metabolism, January 10, 2017, https://www.endocrine.org/news-and-advocacy/news-room/2017/landmark-study-defines-normal-ranges-for-testosterone-levels.

338 Endocrine Society, "New Defined Reference Range."

Printed in the USA
CPSIA information can be obtained
at www.ICGtesting.com
JSHW021920080224
56871JS00009B/28/J